AIDS

The Story of
a Disease

AIDS

The Story of a Disease

JOHN GREEN AND
DAVID MILLER

GRAFTON BOOKS
A Division of the Collins Publishing Group

LONDON GLASGOW
TORONTO SYDNEY AUCKLAND

Grafton Books
A Division of the Collins Publishing Group
8 Grafton Street, London W1X 3LA

Published by Grafton Books 1986

British Library Cataloguing in Publication Data

Green, John
    AIDS: the story of a disease.
    1. AIDS (Disease)
    I. Title   II. Miller, David, 1955–
    616.9'792   RC607.A26

    ISBN 0-246-12982-4

Photoset by Rowland Phototypesetting Ltd,
Bury St Edmunds, Suffolk
Printed in Great Britain by
William Collins Sons & Co. Ltd, Glasgow

CONTENTS

ACKNOWLEDGEMENTS

The authors would like to thank many people for the part they played in enabling us to write this book, in particular Dr Don Jeffries, Dr Susan Forster, Heather George, Geraldine Mulleady and Alana McCreaner who provided invaluable advice on the technicalities of a complicated field. If there is any merit in the book it is in large part through their help: any mistakes, we fear, are those of the authors.

We would also like to thank all those who have helped indirectly through useful discussions and helpful advice about issues in AIDS during our day-to-day work. So many people have helped that it would be impossible to mention them all without the book's looking like a telephone directory, but they know who they are and we thank them all. We would especially like to mention Dr Tony Pinching and Mary B. Anthony, Jon Grimshaw and David Kavanagh, Body Positive and the Terrence Higgins Trust, and Lydia Temoshok for her invaluable information about the situation in the United States. Needless to say, the opinions given in this book are our own and not necessarily theirs.

Finally we would like to thank our patients, without whom this book could not have been written. We have learned more from our patients than they have from us.

John Green and David Miller
St Mary's Hospital, London
February 1986

NOTE

There is still disagreement amongst scientists as to what the virus which can cause AIDS should be called. In America it is called HTLV-III, in France LAV. In this book, for the sake of consistency we have called it HTLV-III, the name it is most often known by in the English-speaking world.

NB: Since the time of writing, the official designation for the AIDS virus has changed from HTLV-III to HIV (Human Immunodeficiency Virus).

INTRODUCTION

I* remember very well the first time that I saw an AIDS patient, in 1983. He was one of the very earliest cases in the UK. I had been called to see him because he had just come in and was not only worried about his condition but also felt, wrongly as it turned out, that his memory and ability to think had been affected.

It was a wet, miserable day and the hospital looked particularly gloomy. I put on a mask, gloves and an apron and went to see him. This was early in the epidemic, and we had just found out that the disease could be transmitted but were not sure how easily it was transmitted or in what ways. These days we take none of these precautions simply to go and talk to a patient: they are just not necessary.

He was sitting in his room watching children's programmes on the television. He looked fairly cheerful and clearly regarded his condition as something of a novelty.

'I'll bet you've never seen anything quite like this,' he said, and drew the bedclothes off his feet. 'Kaposi's sarcoma. Everyone I've shown it to is fascinated by it.'

His feet were covered in a purplish mass of skin tumour, far more than I have ever seen since. It looked just as though he had dipped his feet into a bowl full of blueberries and the skin

* John Green

11

had been stained. Kaposi's sarcoma is so rare in people who do not have AIDS that I had never seen it before. We both stared at it; he was more interested than concerned.

Then he told me the story of his life. A gay man, he had a job which was not very well paid. A couple of years before he had finally managed to save up for what he described, wrily, as the holiday of a lifetime.. He went to San Francisco where he had a good time and had sex with a small number of American men. This was at a time when AIDS was only just being recognised in America. One of the men was probably infected with the virus that causes AIDS.

After a while he was discharged home. Somehow the newspapers had found out about him, probably through one of the people he had told. He woke up one morning to find his garden full of newspapermen, including a cameraman hiding in the bushes. Only threats of legal action from the hospital dissuaded them from their macabre vigil.

Over the next few months I saw him a number of times. Conversation was easier without the mask and shaking hands more natural without the gloves. Unfortunately, although treatment was causing the Kaposi's sarcoma on his foot to regress somewhat, new patches of tumour were appearing elsewhere, including his stomach. Eventually he died. He died because his body had no defence against disease and no defence against the tumour which it would normally not have allowed to develop.

Since then the authors of this book have seen over a hundred people with AIDS. Some of them have had AIDS since 1983 and are still apparently in reasonably good health. At the same time we have seen many hundreds of people who do not have AIDS but are infected with the virus which causes it, HTLV-III.

In 1985 we began a series of weekend workshops aimed at health professionals, doctors, nurses, social workers, health advisers, psychologists and others who were working with this

disease. The workshops eventually became a national resource for training funded by the Department of Health.
Through the workshops and through our research work we
have had the opportunity to meet many of the people working
in this field not just in the UK but abroad. Their experiences
have been valuable in helping us to understand the problem.

This book is aimed at all those who are interested in AIDS.
It is aimed at those who work in hospitals, who may come
into contact with the problem sooner or later and want a
non-technical guide, and at those who feel they may be at
risk; most of all it is aimed at those people who do not have
any direct involvement in the problem but who want to know
more about the fascinating story of the disease which has
been called 'the greatest threat to health since the Second
World War'.

Chapter One

THE STORY OF
A DISEASE

The story of AIDS starts at the Centers for Disease Control in
Atlanta, Georgia. The job of the CDC is to monitor infectious and other diseases in the United States, such as gonorrhoea, hepatitis, mumps and typhoid, and to publish information on the spread and treatment of these illnesses in its
journal, sombrely entitled *Morbidity and Mortality Weekly
Report (MMWR)*.

In 1981 the CDC began to receive reports of the appearance in young men of cases of a chest infection called
pneumocystis carinii pneumonia (PCP). PCP is caused by a
parasite which the body's defences against disease, the immune system, are usually able to keep under control. In
adults it rarely causes disease. After the last war cases were
common in prisoners released from concentration camps,
and cases still occur in areas of the world where nutrition
is poor and so people are less able to fight disease. However, these considerations did not apply to the cases being
reported, nor did the people who were getting PCP seem
to fit into any of the other known risk categories. The
CDC was soon on the scent of a trail that it pursues to this
day.

At the same time that the CDC were becoming concerned
about the increase in PCP they began to receive reports of
something else that didn't seem to add up. Physicians were

beginning to report large numbers of young men coming to them with a rare skin tumour, Kaposi's sarcoma (KS). This usually attacks only elderly men of Jewish or Mediterranean origin. It is also sometimes seen in people whose immune systems have been depressed, for instance by the drugs used to prevent rejection of organ transplants. It was very unusual in young men with none of the usual risk factors.

The link between PCP and Kaposi's sarcoma seemed to be that they both occur most often in people whose immune systems are weakened in some way, by drugs, by malnutrition or by age. None of these things applied to the cases reported to the CDC, but there was one thing that linked them: all the cases were homosexual men.

The first report of these cases of PCP, Kaposi's sarcoma and some other rare infections appeared in *Morbidity and Mortality Weekly Report* on 5 June 1981. It seemed that a new illness was appearing in the country and it was particularly affecting homosexual men.

In order to assess the impact of these baffling new illnesses associated with immune deficiencies, the CDC set up a task force to keep track of the growing number of cases and try to assess those most likely to be at risk. While the progress of PCP in the population was monitored, the appearance of the other illnesses associated with immune deficiency was also monitored by written and telephoned reports from doctors around the country. Shortly afterwards, the Communicable Disease Surveillance Centre (CDSC) of the Public Health Laboratory Service in London started collecting statistics on the appearance of such illnesses in England. The mystery killer had by now been given a new name: Acquired Immune Deficiency Syndrome (AIDS). For the purposes of its surveillance, the CDC defined the condition:

1. Patients having a reliably diagnosed disease (such as pneumocystis carinii pneumonia or Kaposi's sarcoma in a

person less than 60 years of age) suggestive of an underlying cellular immune defect;
2. The disease occurs in the absence of a cellular immune
   deficiency that could be due to other factors (e.g. use of
   immunosuppressive drugs or the presence of a lympho-
   reticular malignancy).

At the time it was formulated, this definition was criticised for
being both too restrictive and too broad, but it did prove
extraordinarily useful in providing a helpful analysis of those
groups and individuals who were at risk of catching AIDS.

About a year after the initial reports, reports began to
appear of similar cases in Haitian immigrants to the United
States and in haemophiliacs. This added a new dimension to
the drama of the emerging epidemic. As the roll of fatalities
unwound, revealing more categories of patients – those
receiving blood transfusions, infants, female sexual partners
of men in other risk groups, intravenous (heroin-injecting)
drug abusers – it became clear that those groups of persons
who had fallen victim to the disease shared two major links:
sex and/or blood. As the agent responsible for the development of AIDS had yet to be identified, epidemiologists in
America began to investigate the life-styles of the patient
group – male homosexuals – in an attempt to see whether the
pattern of sexual activity of gay men was somehow involved
in the appearance of AIDS.

One early study, involving 50 gay men with AIDS and 120
matched gay men without AIDS, found that the development of AIDS was most strongly associated with higher
numbers of sexual partners than for non-AIDS controls
(roughly twice the number – an average of around 60 per
year). Other factors associated with the development of AIDS
included starting regular anal intercourse at an earlier age
than non-patients, greater exposure (oral and anal) to faeces
(in reality more anal and anal–oral sex), a higher exposure to

syphilis and non-B hepatitis, and a longer use of nitrites, a recreational drug much used by gay men, than non-patients.

This information was particularly useful, because it provided evidence relating specific behaviours in homosexual men to their risk of getting AIDS. It did not, unfortunately, tell what was causing AIDS itself, although much time was spent speculating on why such behaviour should make AIDS more likely. For instance, the possibility of repeated tearing of the rectum during anal intercourse, together with repeated exposure to faeces and sexually transmitted infections (as would be much more likely with higher numbers of casual sexual partners), all in the context of a high rate of usage of nitrites as sexual stimulants, led to the development of a theory of the development of AIDS variously called the 'hot-bed' or 'immune overload' theory.

This theory proposed that T lymphocytes, a group of cells vital to the body's defences against disease, were being subjected to enormous strain by repeated infection and chemical damage from nitrites, resulting in an eventual irreversible degree of damage, AIDS. It was unclear how this suggested mechanism alone could account for the clinical picture seen in AIDS patients, but it did seem plausible that the repeated sexually transmitted infections reported in patients, which could themselves mildly depress the immune system, could play a significant part in the development of the syndrome.

Some investigators focused on sperm itself as the main problem. Where homosexual men were having high rates of anal intercourse they might be receiving significant amounts of sperm which would infiltrate the blood stream through tears in the rectum. It was thought possible that the immune system could be damaged directly by the sperm. Results from mice showed that very large amounts of sperm getting into the bloodstream could indeed suppress the immune system, but the amounts of sperm involved in these experiments were

18

very large, more than would be expected to get into the bloodstream in anal intercourse.

A similar theory about the cause of AIDS focused on the high rate of recreational drug abuse in patients. Extensive use of nitrites (inhaled to heighten and prolong the effects of sexual arousal and orgasm) had been well documented in homosexual patients, and it was thought that this element alone could possibly account for the destruction of immune efficiency. However, closer investigation revealed that even prolonged use of such chemicals did not produce immune effects of the order that would be required for irreversible immune damage. Moreover, many people seemed to make heavy use of nitrites with no apparent ill-effects. An important observation was, however, made concerning the high correlation of drug usage with large numbers of sexual partners: when people are drugged or drunk, their motivation for casual sexual activity increases, leading to more frequent and variable sexual behaviour.

The logic of the growing epidemic, by now involving almost all the states in America – and many countries in Europe – suggested that a third theory might provide the answer. Some sort of infection might be involved. This suggestion received backing from the discovery that some of the homosexual men who were getting AIDS had had sex with one another. Perhaps they were passing on some sort of infectious agent? But what agent?

The spread of AIDS among homosexual men indicated that such an agent would be capable of being spread sexually, perhaps by exposure to blood during anal intercourse from minute tearing of the thin lining of the rectum. The emergence of AIDS in haemophiliac patients suggested that the agent could be passed on through Factor VIII concentrate, a blood-clotting agent used in the treatment of haemophilia, which is prepared from large pools of blood donors. It seemed possible that some of these donors could have been infected with the virus without knowing it, and it appeared conceivable that they could have passed on the infectious agent by this means.

It was also becoming clear that many injecting drug addicts were developing the syndrome. The American facility of 'shooting galleries', where addicts hire syringes to inject drugs, had long been implicated in the wide spread of infectious agents. The syringes hired in such places are not sterilised and are shared by many people. It seemed likely that any blood-borne infectious agent responsible for AIDS could be spread very quickly among large numbers of people using the same syringe.

At the same time, cases of AIDS were appearing in groups not previously thought to be at risk. There were cases in the female sexual partners of men in high-risk groups. Vaginal sexual intercourse without any apparent involvement of blood appeared to be a risk factor in the development of AIDS, suggesting that other bodily fluids than blood must contain the agent responsible, particularly semen. Cases were reported in the children of mothers who were intravenous drug abusers, suggesting whatever was causing the disease could be passed on in the womb or at birth.

The ways in which AIDS appeared to be spread all pointed to one sort of infectious agent, a virus. Massive efforts to isolate this virus got under way in the United States, Paris and London.

By this time, cases were rising in America at an exponential rate. The first reports involving five patients with PCP were rapidly followed by reports of KS in 26 young men, then 70 further cases of these two conditions in the next month. By the end of 1981 cases totalled 252 (including hitherto unrecognised cases dating back to 1978). The numbers of patients were doubling every six months, with an average of 4–5 cases being reported to the CDC every day by March 1983. By December 1983 cases totalled 2,643. By April

1985, American cases totalled 10,000, over half of whom had been reported in the previous 12 months. By December 1985, American cases totalled a staggering 15,775 cases in just four years. Of all the reported cases 49% of the adults and 69% of the children had died, and roughly 75% of all those diagnosed before 1983 had died from their illnesses. From the earliest days of reporting until mid-1983, most American cases were in the large cities on the east, west and south coasts (New York, San Francisco, Los Angeles and Miami). Cases then began appearing in greater numbers from other American centres. Today all American states have reported AIDS cases, as the disease has spread from large cities to rural areas and small towns.

In England the same exponential development in case numbers has been seen, although the numbers have been smaller. The first cases (three) appeared in 1982. In 1983 there were 28 reported, in 1984 there were 71, and in 1985 there were 167. The total number of cases in the United Kingdom on 31 December 1985 was 265, of whom 140 had died. The American experience of an early appearance in the larger urban areas (London) has been repeated.

In the search for an infectious agent that might be the cause of AIDS, the logical first step was to review those viruses known to cause severe illness which could be passed in blood and semen. The continuing analysis of cases reported to doctors the world over helped to exclude a number of virus types, making the focus sharper. For example, there were no known cases of AIDS in health workers in close proximity to patients, suggesting that the agent was not airborne and that contact with intact skin was not a way in which the virus could be passed on.

Suspect viruses were vetted thoroughly, but with little early success. A virus called cytomegalovirus (CMV) was found in all the patients who had been the subject of the first reports of PCP in the *MMWR*. CMV has for many years been found very frequently among homosexual men attending sexually transmitted disease clinics – one notable study in 1981 found CMV in 94% of homosexual clinic attenders. Researchers had also found infectious CMV in semen, suggesting that it could be sexually transmitted. A further clue to CMV as the possible agent in AIDS was its known association with cellular immunosuppressive states, its isolation from tissue cultures of Kaposi's sarcoma, and similarities in the immunological abnormalities seen in both AIDS and CMV infection.

Despite the suggestions pointing to CMV as the cause, other evidence suggested otherwise. In particular, CMV was not often found in heterosexual AIDS patients and it has been around for a long time – if it were the cause, AIDS on the present scale would have been expected to have occurred before now. On the other hand, it was at least possible that the virus might have mutated in some way to produce AIDS. Similar considerations applied to a relative of CMV, Epstein-Barr virus, which also came under suspicion. Another suspect virus was hepatitis B virus (HBV). Although this agent is commonly found in people with AIDS, it is not found in all, and therefore it, like CMV, did not appear to be the cause.

A potential candidate that excited early interest was African swine fever virus (ASFV), which had been found to infect wild pigs in Africa. Soon after its discovery it was isolated in African domestic pigs. The virus is also found in Europe, Latin America and the Caribbean (including Haiti). Infected pigs suffer immune abnormalities similar to those seen in human AIDS patients, together with anorexia and fever. One researcher hypothesised that this virus may have passed from pigs to man by a homosexual Haitian eating pork infected with ASFV. The virus could have entered his bloodstream through a stomach abscess or ulcer and could then have been passed onto sexual contacts. Despite this idea there was no evidence that ASFV infection caused AIDS.

While researchers were attempting to complete the causative jigsaw with these possible answers, research was going on into other promising lines of enquiry. One that looked particularly promising was a rather strange family of viruses, the retroviruses. Such viruses were unknown in humans before 1980, though several animal retroviruses had already been identified. There were only two retroviruses known to affect humans, HTLV-I, which was known to cause leukaemia, and HTLV-II, which did not appear to be directly implicated in any known human disease, but did have many similarities with HTLV-I.

The possibility that a human retrovirus might be the agent responsible for AIDS was supported by the observation that an animal retrovirus, feline leukaemia virus, caused AIDS-like immune destruction in wild cats. One recent study in the light of the AIDS epidemic revealed that up to 90% of feral cats in parts of Glasgow are infected with this virus. It cannot be passed on to people, but it provided an example of a virus causing something that looked like AIDS in an animal.

In 1983 the pace quickened. Antibodies to HTLV-I were identified in blood from roughly 40% of AIDS patients studied by a research team at Harvard in America. However, these antibodies related to the membrane or 'envelope' surrounding the known HTLV viruses, not to the known internal structures of these retroviruses. Further, such antibodies were not found in the blood of all the patients analysed – perhaps another undiscovered member of this strange virus family was responsible. If this was sufficiently similar to HTLV-I there might be 'cross reactivity', that is, antibodies to one virus might react in some cases with the other virus.

Between late 1982 and early 1983 a new retrovirus had been isolated in a number of different centres in the United States, but any certain characterisation of this novel agent was frustrated by an inability either to reproduce transmissions of the virus to other cells or to 'grow' them reliably on a sufficient scale to compare these virus isolates with one another. It was not possible to tell whether these reports concerned the same virus, nor, if it was the same virus, whether it was responsible for AIDS.

Then a vital breakthrough came. A team of doctors at the Pasteur Institute in Paris reported in mid-1983 that they had isolated a new retrovirus, called lymphadenopathy-associated virus (LAV), that was distinct from the other known human retroviruses and which had been identified in a male homosexual with persistent generalised lymphadeno-pathy (PGL – considered at that time to be an indicator of the eventual onset of AIDS). Shortly afterwards Robert Gallo in the United States reported that he had isolated a similar virus from some samples he had been working on which he called HTLV-III. At last the virus had been reliably characterised. The next hurdle was to find a way of growing it and testing its activity in target cells. The report heralding that this final obstacle had been overcome came in 1984: from then on it was possible to identify specifically a retrovirus that was linked to the development of AIDS, and to do so reliably. The initial and subsequent investigations on the blood from AIDS patients, as well as those with 'pre-AIDS' symptoms, confirmed that HTLV-III was indeed the causative agent.

The battle to identify the enemy had been won, and in a remarkably short time. It is sobering to consider that even five years earlier the identification of HTLV-III might not have been possible. No human retroviruses were known and the methods needed to culture HTLV-III were not available. Fifteen years earlier animal retroviruses were unknown. If AIDS had appeared at that time, medical science would have been a helpless bystander as the epidemic raged.

Once having identified the probable virus, the next steps were to involve teasing apart this new viral intruder so that its point of weakness could be found and, in turn, attacked, then finding a means of easily identifying the virus in the populations at risk so that effective steps could be taken to reduce and, if possible, halt its further spread.

Since the early cases AIDS has become the number one priority in health for many governments. Cases are no longer restricted to gay men, haemophiliacs and intravenous drug abusers, although they still bear the main brunt of this terrible disease. And it has become clear that AIDS is not limited to America and Europe: it is causing a massive epidemic in Africa, where heterosexuals are the main risk group. The story of the attempts to stop the spread and to find a cure is the subject of the rest of this book.

Chapter Two

THE VIRUS

AIDS is caused by a virus, HTLV-III. Viruses are very simple objects indeed, really little more than packets of chemicals whose only purpose is to reproduce themselves. They can reproduce themselves only by invading the cells of an animal or plant and using those cells for their own ends.

Around the outside of the HTLV-III virus particle is a membrane. This membrane is a few millionths of an inch thick and is made up of protein, which the virus makes itself, and a fatty material which it steals from the cells of its host. It is as though it were wrapped in the thinnest possible coat of butter. It is this membrane which makes the AIDS virus so sensitive. Detergents such as ordinary washing-up liquid, bleach, dry-cleaning fluid and a whole host of everyday chemicals will destroy the membrane. If it is heated the virus is destroyed.

Inside the virus particle is the genome. This contains the basic information the virus needs to reproduce itself.

At the heart of every cell is a complex chain of chemicals called deoxyribonucleic acid (DNA). It looks like two springs coiled tightly around each other. Each spring is actually made up of a chain of thousands of bases. These are very simple chemicals, and in fact there are only four of them in DNA, adenine (A), guanine (G), cytosine (C) and thymine (T).

DNA is the blueprint of the cell. The bases can spell out millions of different messages, just as the dots and dashes of Morse code can spell out thousands of words. But the bases spell out not words but chemical formulae. When the cell requires any particular chemical to continue its work the formula is contained somewhere within its DNA. It is only necessary for it to activate the right part of the DNA chain and the chemical can be made.

DNA makes the chemicals it needs by manufacturing another rather similar chemical called ribonucleic acid (RNA). The RNA then moves out into the body of the cell away from the DNA and attracts the bits and pieces it needs to make whatever chemical it requires. It is rather as though a half-completed jigsaw (the RNA) were able to move through a box of jigsaw pieces (various chemicals in the cell) and attract the bits it needed. As it collected the pieces it would slot them together so that they in turn were linked to each other. That is exactly what RNA does. It assembles complex chemicals out of simple components.

The way in which HTLV-III works is best seen by looking at another virus, the herpes virus, cause of cold sores around the mouth as well as the sexually transmitted disease herpes. This virus is a DNA virus, that is, its genome is made up of DNA just like that in the cells of the person that it infects. Once the virus gets inside a cell in a person's body it slots its own DNA into the DNA of that cell by breaking the DNA chain of the cell, inserting itself and then connecting up to the two broken ends. The virus becomes a part of the cell's own blueprint. It then switches on that part of the DNA, but instead of making chemicals that the cell needs it begins to make copies of the virus. These copies of the virus escape from the cell and infect other cells, which are also turned over to making copies of the virus which go on to infect other cells, and so on.

HTLV-III is, however, a much more complicated virus

27

than herpes. It is part of a group of viruses which are called the retroviruses, because they work in the opposite way to the rest of nature. DNA achieves its ends by making RNA. In nature RNA never makes DNA – except in retroviruses.

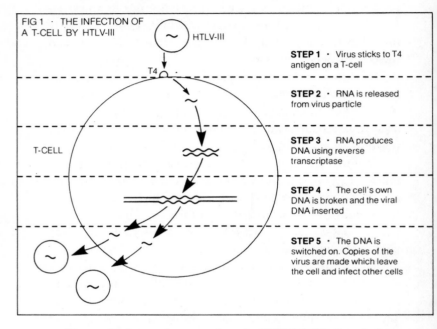

FIG 1 · THE INFECTION OF A T-CELL BY HTLV-III

HTLV-III

T4

T-CELL

STEP 1 · Virus sticks to T4 antigen on a T-cell

STEP 2 · RNA is released from virus particle

STEP 3 · RNA produces DNA using reverse transcriptase

STEP 4 · The cell's own DNA is broken and the viral DNA inserted

STEP 5 · The DNA is switched on. Copies of the virus are made which leave the cell and infect other cells

Figure 1 shows the way that the HTLV-III virus infects cells. It is most likely to attack a sort of cell called a T-cell, of which more later. It actually attacks the T-cell by sticking to a special receptor on the surface called the T4 antigen. The T-cell possesses this receptor for other purposes, enabling the T-cell to carry out some special task. It seems likely that the T-cell mistakes the virus for something else and so lets it in, or that the virus has adapted to this receptor. Once inside the cell the virus rapidly sheds its coat.

Inside the virus, when it has lost its coat, is a single strand of RNA. The RNA builds a double-stranded section of DNA, inserts this DNA into the DNA of the cell, takes over the cell and starts making copies of the virus. This is a very unusual process indeed. RNA is actually making DNA. In order to do so the virus has to produce a special chemical called reverse transcriptase (RNA dependent DNA polymerase). Because nothing else in nature makes DNA from RNA, nothing else in nature produces reverse transcriptase. If a drug could be found which would destroy reverse transcriptase but do nothing else, it would prevent the virus working without harming the person taking the drug.

The retroviruses are a complete family of viruses. They were first properly characterised in 1970. They cause a large number of diseases in animals, particularly different sorts of cancer. For instance, they cause leukaemia (blood cancer) and sarcomas (tumours of the supportive tissues of the body) in mice and chickens. They have now been recognised to cause a whole range of diseases other than cancer.

One particularly interesting retrovorus is the cat leukaemia virus, sometimes called 'feline AIDS virus', although it is not a close relative of HTLV-III. This has only recently been recognised as one of the greatest causes of death in the adult domestic cat. It causes not just leukaemia but also an AIDS-like syndrome in which the cat becomes prey to a whole host of infections. It also directly causes all sorts of illnesses in cats which are only beginning to be recognised. What makes it so interesting is that it has been possible to develop a prototype vaccine which protects cats against the effects of this virus. This gives some hope of developing a similar vaccine against HTLV-III, although the feline virus is more stable genetically than HTLV-III and produces neutralising antibody, so that the analogy cannot be taken too far. Needless to say, the cat leukaemia virus cannot be passed on to people.

It was only in the mid-seventies that a retrovirus was found in man. This virus was called HTLV-I, the Human T-cell

Leukaemia Virus, and it seems to be a relative of HTLV-III, although a fairly distant one.

It has long been known that a certain type of leukaemia tends to be found in certain geographical areas, in the southern states of North America, in Central Africa and, most particularly, on the southern islands of Japan. This disease tends to cluster in families and evidence appeared that it could be passed on not just from parent to child but also sexually and through blood transfusion. Eventually it was found to be caused by the HTLV-I retrovirus. This discovery was difficult to make because until recently the T-cells could not be made to multiply outside the body. It was only when this could be achieved that it was possible to make enough cells to manufacture sufficient virus to identify it.

The strange thing about HTLV-I is that it has an incubation period of up to 40 years. That is, from actually getting the virus to the appearance of leukaemia takes up to half a lifetime. Moreover, only one person in every hundred infected with the virus will actually develop leukaemia. The other 99 are apparently quite unaffected by their unwelcome visitor.

More recently a second member of the family, HTLV-II, has been identified. It was isolated from two cases of 'hairy-cell' leukaemia. However, it did not seem that it was actually causing the leukaemia; something else was, and the virus was probably a chance finding in these patients. At the moment HTLV-II is a virus without a disease – at least we do not know what disease it causes, if it causes one at all. Some viruses seem to cause no disease, and possibly HTLV-II is one of them. But we may be in for a nasty surprise in years to come. There is evidence that HTLV-I and HTLV-II may be spreading through the homosexual population of North America. There are no signs at the moment that they are causing widespread disease, but the future cannot be predicted. Like

HTLV-III they seem to be sexually transmitted or passed on from parent to child.

It is of course possible that there are many retroviruses which have yet to be discovered. They may hold the key to many of the diseases which puzzle modern medicine.

There is some reason to suppose that the three HTLV viruses are rather distant relatives. There is no evidence that HTLV-III causes leukaemia, or indeed any other cancer; indeed, there is good evidence that it works in the opposite way to these other viruses. HTLV-I causes T-cells to multiply and to become immortal, HTLV-III kills T-cells. The relatives of HTLV-III will be covered in more detail in Chapter 5.

THE IMMUNE SYSTEM

The body has a vast array of defences against disease which are known collectively as the immune system. HTLV-III attacks this system directly and undermines its efficiency. By doing so it makes the infected person vulnerable to disease. To be precise, it makes some people vulnerable: in others the virus seems to have little effect. Why this should be so is a puzzle.

The body has many lines of defence against a virus like HTLV-III. The first line of defence is the skin. This is a tough, dry barrier, inhospitable to most disease organisms. If HTLV-III gets on to intact skin it is unable to enter the body and it soon dies. That is one reason why there is no risk of infection with HTLV-III through casual contact, by shaking hands for instance.

Not all parts of the body exposed to the environment are actually covered in skin. The linings of the nose and mouth, the genitals, the inside of the lungs and the rectum, are covered in moist soft tissue. These tissues are protected by a variety of chemicals which defend them against invasion and usually protect against infection. Even so, it is through these surfaces that most disease-causing organisms pass. Because HTLV-III is not an airborne virus like the common cold, the surfaces it usually attacks are those of the genitals and rectum. The other route by which it can get into the body is if it is injected, as in blood transfusions with infected blood or by 'needle-stick injuries', where a doctor or nurse taking a blood sample is punctured by the needle.

Even where there is a needle-stick injury, the chances of someone being infected with the disease are very low. The reason is straightforward. Although in theory a single virus particle can lead to disease, in real life a certain amount of virus is required. One reason for this may be because a special type of cell, a phagocyte (eating cell), which circulates in the bloodstream, attacks foreign material and engulfs it before it can cause disease. If only a minute amount of virus enters the body, it is unlikely that any of it will escape the phagocytes to reach other body cells and infect them.

The next line of defence by the body is the adaptive immune system. The barrier systems described above always work in exactly the same way. If you encounter measles virus several times in your life these systems respond in exactly the same way each time, neither better nor worse. They are fixed, they do not learn. But if you are exposed to measles virus several times in your life you usually become ill only the first time. That is because the adaptive immune system recognises the second time round that it has encountered measles virus before, and it is able to mount a much more effective attack on the virus. The adaptive immune system has learned how to deal with measles virus. Once the virus enters the body some virus particles are picked up by cells called antigen-presenting cells. Their job is to show the virus particle to other parts of the immune system which will actually find a way to destroy it.

An antigen is anything that the body recognises as foreign. In practice, the body does not recognise the whole of the virus as foreign, but several different parts of it. This means that an attack can be mounted even when the body sees only a bit of the virus, something very important for reasons discussed later.

The antigen-presenting cells present the virus to a special group of cells called B-cells. There are enormous numbers of B-cells in the blood and there seem to be up to 100 million different types of B-cell. Each different type carries chemicals on its surface which will stick to only one type of antigen. These chemicals which stick to antigens are called antibodies. It seems that the average adult possesses at birth or soon after antibodies to every single disease they could ever encounter and even to chemicals which do not exist in nature.

The antigen-presenting cell presents the virus particle to every B-cell it can find. At some point it will find a B-cell which is carrying antibodies that will stick to the virus, or part of the virus. As soon as it is found, the B-cell will start to reproduce itself at an enormous rate, pumping out copies of the antibodies it has on its surface into the circulation. These will stick to virus particles in the bloodstream. As soon as they stick they attract all sorts of cells which engulf and destroy the virus. They also cause special complement chemicals to become active and destroy the virus particle.

Here is where the importance of the fact that it is bits of the virus which are attacked comes in. When HTLV-III reproduces itself it does so within the cells of the human body. This means that the antibody cannot get at the virus, which is protected by the cell it is existing in. However, when viruses are reproducing in a cell bits of them actually appear studded in the outside wall of the cell. Antibodies fasten on to these bits. This means that antibodies not only stick to virus itself, they also stick to cells which have been infected with virus.

33

The antibodies then attract chemicals and cells which kill the infected cell and so the virus that it contains.

In order for B-cells to produce antibodies they need help, in most cases, from T-cells producing chemicals called lymphokines which help the B-cells to recognise foreign materials and to start to produce antibodies. These 'helper cells' are the ones which are particularly prone to infection with HTLV-III. The virus invades them and kills some of them. It also seems to be able to make helper cells less effective, even those which are not actually infected with the virus. The result is that in AIDS the patient's body fails to produce specific antibodies to fight disease as it should.

Some T-cells are themselves able directly to attack virus-infected cells without antibodies being involved. These cyto-toxic (cell-killing) T-cells do not function properly in AIDS, although they are not themselves directly infected.

The lack of antibodies and the defects in cell-killing T-cells leaves patients wide open to all sorts of infections which their bodies would normally fight off.

THE ANTIBODY TEST

When a person is infected with HTLV-III the body produces antibodies to that particular virus. The problem with these antibodies is that they are not 'neutralising'. This simply means that they fail to cause the destruction of the virus, or the cells which contain the virus. The antibodies stick to virus or to bits of virus studded in the cell wall, but then things go wrong: they do not attract the all-out assault from the immune system that one would expect. Solving the puzzle of why they do not could provide some key answers to the enigma of AIDS.

In fact, someone infected with HTLV-III produces not just one type of antibody but several against different bits of the virus. Some people seem to produce some neutralising antibody to the virus, but not necessarily enough to be effective, and it looks as though other people produce none or very little. Again, locating antibodies which do neutralise the virus, which cause it and the cells which contain it to be attacked, is a very important area of research. If it were possible to obtain neutralising antibody it might be feasible to make it in the laboratory and so to attack the virus artificially.

The presence of antibodies to the virus does, however, have one interesting use. It allows people to find out whether they have been infected with the virus. There are several different ways of finding out whether someone has antibodies to the virus. One of these tests is known as the Elisa. The test is complicated, and it is unnecessary to know about it in detail in order to understand it, but this, in outline, is how one type of Elisa works:

Bits of virus (viral antigens) are stuck to the walls of plastic dishes. The patient's blood is then put into the dishes. Naturally, if there are antibodies to HTLV-III present they will stick to the bits of virus. The next step is to wash away the excess blood. Then a second set of antibodies is added. These are special antibodies made by injecting human antibodies into animals. In these circumstances the animal produces antibodies to human antibodies, known as anti-human-immunoglobulins (immunoglobulin is another word for antibody). We can call them anti-antibodies.

If there are antibodies stuck to the virus the anti-antibodies will stick to them. The anti-antibodies have been specially treated with a chemical which we can call chemical A. Again everything is washed out so that only anti-antibodies actually stuck to something remain. The next step is to add chemical B, which changes colour in the presence of chemical A. If there is a colour change it means that there must be anti-antibodies present. If anti-antibodies are present, specific antibodies to the virus must be present. If there are specific antibodies, then the person must have been infected with HTLV-III.

At present we believe that anyone who has ever been infected with HTLV-III stays infected with the virus: antibodies stay in their blood. The only exception is really ill AIDS patients who appear to have no antibodies to the virus in some cases. It is probable that they are simply not producing sufficient antibodies to be detected by most of the tests in common use. Because of immune system damage, antibody production in such patients may be severely reduced.

Not only do we believe that anyone infected with the virus stays infected, but that most if not all people infected with the virus remain infectious to others. This is because their cells are continuously releasing fresh virus. If there are people who are not infectious to others we have no way yet of recognising who they are.

The important things to remember about the test are these:

● It does not show that someone has AIDS, only that the person has been infected with the virus at one time or another.

● It does not show that someone will develop AIDS in the future.

● It sometimes makes mistakes, like any other test. Perhaps 25 tests in every 100,000 appear to show that the virus is present when in fact it is not. That is a low failure rate by any standards, but still rather too high for comfort. More worrying still, some people infected with the virus seem to show no antibodies at all, perhaps as many as 4% of people infected with the virus. Why this should be so no one knows. That is one of the reasons why people in high-risk groups should never give blood even after a blood test that is negative (shows up no antibodies).

THE GENOME

The genome of the virus is the blueprint it uses to make copies of itself. This blueprint is made up of a series of bases which spell out various chemical formulae to make whatever the virus needs to reproduce itself. If we consider the chemical formulae as words, then the genome of the virus can be considered as made up of a series of sentences, each of which spells out the complete make-up of a particular part of the virus, for instance its membrane, the coat it wears. These sentences are called genes.

The genomes of human beings are also made up of genes. There are genes which specify what colour your eyes or hair will be, how tall you will grow and how resistant your teeth will be to decay. Usually in people several genes are needed for complicated things such as height. In viruses usually only one gene specifies one part of the virus.

FIG 2 · THE MAIN GENES ON
THE GENOME OF HTLV-III

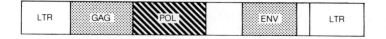

Figure 2 shows the genome of HTLV-III. In fact there are at least two more small genes in the genome of HTLV-III but we are unsure what they do. They may help to make the virus so active. However, we do know the purposes of the main genes. These are called 'gag' (which makes the specific proteins the virus contains), 'pol' (which makes the reverse transcriptase the virus needs to perform the trick of making DNA from RNA) and 'env' (which makes the envelope of the virus). The parts marked LTR at each end of the genome are called 'long terminal repeats' and their purpose is to slot the virus into the genome of the cell it has invaded and to switch it on.

Every example of HTLV-III isolated from different patients has this same structure. However, when you look more closely at the genes from different examples of HTLV-III a rather worrying fact emerges. Within the 'sentence' formed by each gene the actual order of the words differs quite markedly from sample to sample. The virus is highly variable and it is changing and evolving at a high rate. This makes it extremely difficult to produce a vaccine against the virus. A vaccine is usually effective against only one type of virus. The more variable a virus is, the less likely a vaccine is to prevent infection.

HTLV-III will never be anything other than a blood-borne and sexually-transmitted virus: it could not change that any more than a horse can become a sheep. But as it evolves it may become better at what it does, that is, at switching off the immune system and at passing sexually from person to person.

The other consequence of HTLV-III's being so variable is very important. It might seem obvious that someone who has caught this virus can have sex with another person who has had it. After all, they are both infected, therefore they are not going to catch it again, are they? However, if a person has caught the virus and managed to keep it from taking over, then catches a different strain of the same virus, illness may develop. The body may have been able to cope with the first strain but not with the second. At the moment this is supposition: we have very little evidence about the exact significance of differences between different isolates of the virus. However, it is a sufficiently strong possibility to make it inadvisable for two people infected with the virus to assume that they will come to no harm by having sex together, other than 'safe sex'.

By understanding something about the virus it is possible to see why finding a cure has been so difficult. It is highly variable. It is able to switch off or damage the immune system, which means that drugs are not aided as usual by the body's own resources. The antibodies to the virus that are produced seem to be often ineffective, as far as we know. The search for ways around these problems is covered in depth in Chapter 12.

Chapter Three

AIDS IN AFRICA

There is currently a major epidemic of AIDS in Central Africa. While in the West the main group affected so far has been homosexual men, in Africa AIDS is mainly a heterosexual disease. In some of the main city hospitals in Central Africa up to 40% of the beds are occupied by patients with HTLV-III related conditions. Even more alarmingly, the numbers of people infected with HTLV-III are rising rapidly. What is not clear is why all this is happening, and why in Africa?

What first attracted the attention of researchers to Africa was the high incidence of the skin tumour Kaposi's sarcoma (KS). KS was first described by the Hungarian dermatologist Moriz Kaposi in 1872. It was very rare in Europe in his time and mostly affected elderly men of Jewish or Mediterranean origin. The tumour progressed slowly, showed only slow spread, and the majority of sufferers died of something else, often old age. This pattern is usually called 'classical' KS.

One of the first things that alerted physicians in America to the existence of AIDS was the appearance of KS in young men, as was described in Chapter 1. KS is a common tumour of AIDS patients and in them is frequently much more aggressive, often progressing rapidly and with a far higher mortality rate than in classical KS. The sort of rapidly progressing KS which some AIDS patients get is often called 'atypical' KS, although with the spread of AIDS it is actually commoner nowadays than the classical type.

Although very rare until recently in Europe, KS has always been common in Africa. As long ago as the early 1960s it was known to make up about 10% of all cancers seen in Central African men. It tends to affect men in their twenties and thirties. Naturally this led researchers to look to Africa to see whether AIDS was causing the problem there.

In fact it turns out that there are two main types of KS in Africa just as there are in the West. Until the late 1970s classical KS was the most common type. Patients with this type of KS are not usually infected with HTLV-III. The second type matches the atypical KS seen in AIDS patients, and most Africans with this have been infected with HTLV-III. This atypical type of KS seems to be increasing very rapidly. Cases before 1980 were rare, but they now form the majority of cases.

The explanation for what is happening would seem to be this. HTLV-III does not cause KS, which may well be the result of another infection: a virus of the herpes group, cytomegalovirus, is a likely candidate. Up to 50% of non-gay men show signs of having been infected with this virus in some parts of Africa. The virus is also very common among gay men (it can be sexually transmitted). Cytomegalovirus infection does not lead to KS in most healthy people. However, when someone is infected with HTLV-III it often damages the immune system, which may allow whatever is causing KS, whether cytomegalovirus or some other factor, to create a tumour. In people who are not infected with HTLV-III, and whose immune systems are intact, the KS is restricted and progresses only slowly, producing classical KS. In those who have damaged immune systems KS gets out of control much more rapidly, producing the picture seen in recent African KS cases and in AIDS patients.

41

It is significant that another group of people who are particularly prone to KS are those whose immune systems have been suppressed by drugs used to prevent the immune system killing organs which have been transplanted. People who have had kidney transplants, for example, are perhaps 150–200 times more likely to develop KS than the population at large (although the tumour is so rare that even this risk is a small one). When immunosuppressive drugs are stopped the tumour sometimes regresses.

If these cases of atypical KS have been appearing only recently in Africa does that mean that AIDS is a new disease there too? A great deal of hard work has gone into trying to find out.

Since as far back as the 1950s researchers have collected and stored sera (blood samples) in Africa. They have been studying a whole range of tropical diseases, although they never expected HTLV-III. The obvious step is to take some of the stored sera and to test them for HTLV-III to discover how early the first cases appeared. It sounds fairly straightforward, but in practice there are a number of problems. One difficulty is that the sera have not always been kept in the best of conditions; they have often been repeatedly thawed out and frozen or simply badly stored. This makes doing delicate tests on them rather a problem. A second difficulty is that African sera are often 'sticky', that is, they give many false results on blood tests, including the one for HTLV-III. This 'stickiness' is probably at least in part the result of infections with tropical diseases, especially malaria. (Malaria and a number of other tropical infections cause a non-specific stimulation of antibody production.)

Everywhere that stored sera have been looked at the picture is the same. The further you go back, the less people have been infected with the virus. With some of the very early sera it is even possible that the tests are picking up not HTLV-III but a similar virus, maybe even the forerunner of

HTLV-III. It is also clear that the number of people infected shot up suddenly in the late 1970s and the 1980s and is building up more and more rapidly with each passing year.

The earliest sera analysed so far were collected in 1959 in Central Africa. These were tested for HTLV-III and only one likely HTLV-III infection and two possibles were found out of 672 sera. This would suggest that the infection was rare in the 1950s, even if it really was HTLV-III which was being detected. Studies of sera collected in the mid-1960s show a small number of people probably infected with HTLV-III, but it still seems to have been uncommon. Two-thirds of sera collected in the West Nile area of Uganda in 1972–3 showed evidence of infection with HTLV-III or with some closely-related virus. This seems a very large proportion and it is possible that it reflects some local pocket of some other retrovirus. Other workers have reported that sera they have looked at have shown signs of small numbers of people infected during the early to mid-1970s.

It seems likely that HTLV-III, or a closely-related virus, has been present in Africa for at least ten years and possibly even longer. This contrasts with results from America. The earliest sera to show HTLV-III there date from 1978, suggesting that it was present in Africa some time before appreciable numbers of people were infected in the US.

Since the late seventies the numbers of people infected with HTLV-III in Africa have shot up. The virus has been spreading particularly rapidly in the 1980s, until today the position in Africa appears increasingly desperate. It has been estimated that as many as 10% of adults in parts of Central Africa may be infected with HTLV-III. The virus is clearly spreading outwards from Central Africa into neighbouring states, into Kenya where one per cent of mothers in Nairobi are infected, into Ghana where around six per cent of adults may be infected, into Uganda and into Senegal.

Surveys of HTLV-III infection in Central Africa present

an interesting picture. Two groups of people tend to be infected, very young children and adults from puberty onwards. Very few children from 5 to 14 are infected. From what we know about the transmission of the virus it seems likely that the very young children are being infected from their mothers, in the womb, at birth or by breast-feeding. The virus is found in the breast milk of infected mothers.

There are two possible reasons for the gap between 5 and 14. Firstly, many infected children die in their first two years of life from AIDS. Others are made more susceptible to the infections which are common in African children and they too die. This would mean that few infected children would survive their early years. Secondly, it may be that the sudden upsurge in HTLV-III infection over the last five years means that only children under that age are likely to be infected to a great extent. If this is the case, a generation of infected African children may be growing up at the moment.

Several reasons have been put forward for why adults tend to contract HTLV-III in Africa. In view of the age at which infection levels start to build up, sexual transmission is an obvious suggestion. However, a number of other suggestions have been put forward and it is useful to bear these in mind when considering the evidence.

The first suggestion is that HTLV-III is spread by insects, with the mosquito as the favourite insect. Many viruses are spread by insects, so many that they even have a name, the arboviruses. Viruses spread by mosquitoes include yellow fever, dengue, Japanese B hepatitis and several viruses which attack the brain. The mosquito picks up the virus by sucking blood from someone infected, then it sucks the blood of someone uninfected and passes on the virus. HTLV-III is much less infectious than most of the arboviruses, and the amount of virus passed on by a single mosquito is fairly low. On the other hand, there are enormous numbers of mosquitoes in Africa and they bite at a very high rate. It is possible to be bitten a hundred times an hour if you are unlucky.

The second suggestion is that contaminated syringes used for injections might be the cause of the problem in Africa. Medical facilities are rather poor in many areas, particularly outside the major cities. Much of the medical work is carried out by unqualified people working in poor conditions, and they tend to inject a lot of drugs, partly at least because their patients have more faith in injections than in oral drugs. Hygiene is poor, sterilising of syringes virtually non-existent and the same syringe may be used on a large number of people. These factors are very similar to those which have caused the virus to spread so rapidly among Western drug addicts.

The third suggestion is that scarification is a main factor. Much folk medicine depends on the cutting of the skin, usually with an unsterilised razor-blade, and the rubbing in of various traditional remedies. Sometimes the cutting of the skin itself is thought to convey some benefit. Some peoples in Central Africa also scarify the skin for ritual or cosmetic reasons. Such scarification might conceivably pass the virus around. It has even been suggested that blood-brotherhood rites might spread the virus.

The only way to evaluate these suggestions about the spread of HTLV-III in Africa is to examine the evidence. Some of the best evidence comes from the work of van der Perre and his co-workers in Rwanda. They looked at the blood of over a thousand Rwandans. First they looked at 258 blood donors. Of those living in the city of Kigali 18% were infected, but of those living in rural areas only 4% were infected. A sample of young adults from Kigali and from a rural area showed that 17.5% of Kigali dwellers were infected but only 3% of rural young adults. Eighteen per cent of hospital workers in Kigali were also infected – just the same proportion as the rest of the population. This shows that HTLV-III infection is commoner in the towns than in rural areas. One would expect that town-dwellers would have much better medical facilities and would be much less likely to practise scarification. Hospital workers, who should have had ready access to modern health care methods, were just as likely to be infected as anyone else.

They also looked at prostitutes in Butare city and found that 88% were infected, compared with only 12% of non-prostitute women. Among the customers of prostitutes 28% were positive compared with 17% of other men.

When they surveyed Rwandan AIDS patients they found that the men had higher numbers of sexual partners and more contact with prostitutes. The women included a high number of unmarried women (relatively unusual in Rwandans of their age) and a high number of prostitutes. A third of the women had a promiscuous male partner. This sort of information points strongly towards HTLV-III being spread sexually in Africa, with prostitutes perhaps playing a considerable part in the spread. There is other evidence that points to the same conclusion.

A study was made of people from Nairobi, Kenya, in 1983. Among prostitutes there, a third of higher social class prostitutes and two-thirds of lower-class prostitutes were infected. The more other sexually-transmitted diseases a prostitute had had, the more likely she was to have HTLV-III. The link between social class, number of sexually transmitted diseases and HTLV-III is probably that lower-class women have to have sex with more men to get a reasonable amount of money, and the more partners you have the more diseases you are likely to get.

Attenders at sexually transmitted diseases clinics were also studied, and 5% of them were found to be infected, compared with 2% of medical personnel. Interestingly, the risk of someone being infected was linked to the countries of origin of the people with whom they had sexual relations, with Central African men presenting the highest risk.

It also seems that the numbers of prostitutes in Africa who are infected has risen quite sharply recently. In 1980 7% of Kenyan prostitutes were found to be positive for HTLV-III, in 1984 the figure was 51%. Of men attending a Nairobi sexually transmitted diseases clinic less than 1% gave a positive test result in 1980; now the figure is 13%.

Prostitutes may be a fairly important factor in the spread of HTLV-III in Africa. Several special social factors may encourage some African men to use prostitutes. In much of Central Africa there is a strong taboo against intercourse between a man and his wife for quite a lengthy period after the birth of a child. Men marry late (a factor in the high rate of usage of prostitutes in nineteenth-century London). There are strong taboos against pre-marital sex: the rate of illegitimate births in much of Central Africa is low. Finally, there is a tendency for men to move to the cities and take paid work, leaving their wives behind to look after their land – farming is traditionally women's work in much of Africa. All these factors mean that a large number of young African men are denied contact with women. That is why many African cities have a lot of prostitutes, and it is probably also a major reason for the rapid spread of HTLV-III in Central Africa. Men are likely to bring back HTLV-III and infect their wives and, through them, their children. Unpaid sex also probably plays some part in the spread of the virus, but the influence of prostitution cannot be overestimated.

It is difficult to compare the usage of prostitutes in Africa with that in the West because of the lack of adequate Western comparison data.

There is no evidence at all that insects spread HTLV-III. If they did we would expect a quite different pattern of spread of the virus, both in terms of the ages of people getting the virus – those aged 5–14 would not be expected to be spared infection – and in terms of the geography of the spread. Ritual scarification and the use of unsterilised syringes may account for some of the cases of HTLV-III infection in Central Africa, but it seems unlikely that they are the main factor. Sex is the main factor.

One other suggestion needs to be laid to rest. It has been suggested that the Central Africans engage in anal inter-course at a very high rate for birth control reasons. Certainly anal intercourse has been used as a way of avoiding concep-tion in a whole range of cultures, including Victorian England and parts of the Mediterranean today, but all the evidence points to anal intercourse being much less common in Africa than in the West, not more. The virus is being spread vaginally.

This review of the evidence from Africa covers what seems to have happened so far. Today an ominous change is occurring: the link between the number of sexual partners and the risk of HTLV-III infection seems to be weakening. The reason is straightforward. The rate of spread of any sexually transmitted disease is related to two factors, the number of people infected with the virus at any one time and the number of sexual partners that they have. The number of people infected determines the risk of any one person being infected. The number of sexual partners determines the number of people they will pass it on to. As the number of people infected rises, the number of sexual partners that people have becomes less important. (This point is covered in more detail in Chapter 7.) The implications of this simple formula are clear. In Africa today the spread is likely to increase in speed rather than slowing down until either steps are taken to slow the spread or the population becomes saturated with the virus. There is little sign that effective steps are being taken in Africa at the moment. Central African governments generally lack the resources to mount major health education campaigns and the problems in mounting such campaigns are even greater than they are in the West. Only the West can provide the resources necessary. Unless such aid is forthcoming the situation in Africa is likely to go from bad to worse.

Chapter Four

THE RANGE OF AIDS

A mistake often made by television and newspaper reporters is the assumption that AIDS and HTLV-III infection are the same thing. They are not. There is a major difference between being infected with the virus which can cause AIDS and AIDS itself. AIDS is the last stage of HTLV-III infection, and on present knowledge only a small proportion of those infected with the virus seem to reach it. People with AIDS represent only the tip of the iceberg of all those who have been infected with the HTLV-III virus. Figure 3 illustrates the range of disease states seen in HTLV-III seropositives,

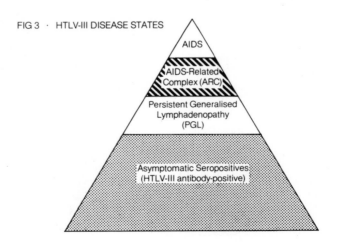

FIG 3 · HTLV-III DISEASE STATES

AIDS

AIDS-Related Complex (ARC)

Persistent Generalised Lymphadenopathy (PGL)

Asymptomatic Seropositives (HTLV-III antibody-positive)

and the relative proportions of those affected. The question of why only a proportion of all those infected actually develop AIDS will be considered later. First it is necessary to consider the different ways in which HTLV-III infection may express itself.

EXPRESSIONS OF HTLV-III INFECTION

1. *Acute retroviral illness*
A patient recently came to St Mary's Hospital asking to be given a full medical examination. This is what he said:

> For the past few days I've had the most awful time. My muscles have been painful. I've been very feverish and shaky, sweating quite heavily and generally feeling unwell – far more so than if I had 'flu, and none of my workmates have had it as usually happens when a bug is about . . .

Close questioning revealed that the patient had, about nine weeks previously, been having sex without the suggested precautions (see Chapter 9) and, as he was homosexual, it seemed possible that his condition was due to acute HTLV-III infection. This sort of reaction is sometimes described as an acute retroviral illness. It usually occurs at about the time that antibodies to the virus appear in the blood, although many people infected with HTLV-III, probably the majority, do not show any signs of this acute illness. They become infected, produce antibodies, but are not aware that they have been infected.

There is no certainty as yet about how long it takes for detectable antibodies to appear in the blood after the virus has entered the patient's bloodstream. The question is an important one, because the blood test for HTLV-III looks for these antibodies and the test will not become positive until they are detectable. It is probable that the time can vary between four

51

weeks and a year or more; however, most people will show antibodies somewhere between 4 and 12 weeks after the virus has entered their system.

How long the symptoms of acute retroviral infection will last, if it occurs at all, is unpredictable. Patients have reported that the symptoms can last from 3–4 days to a couple of weeks. This may well have a great deal to do with the patient's general state of health. After this time, most people feel no further ill-effects. They may remain quite unaware that they have the virus, are 'carriers', and so are infectious to others through blood, semen, organ donations and possibly other bodily fluids. In fact it is thought that up to 70% of infected people have no symptoms or expressions of their infection after antibodies appear. At the moment this conclusion must be a tentative one. The problem with such estimates is that we are as yet only about five years into the HTLV-III epidemic, and there may be long-term effects of infection that have yet to appear.

2. *Persistent Generalised Lymphadenopathy (PGL)*
About 30% of those with HTLV-III infection develop a persistent swelling of their lymph glands (or 'lymphadeno-pathy'). This swelling, which is not usually painful, occurs around the neck, armpits and groin (hence 'generalised'). The lymph glands (properly lymph nodes) may vary in how much they are swollen over time though they do not seem to go down completely. Swollen lymph nodes are common in many infections and the swelling has to be present for at least three months before a diagnosis of PGL can be made.

Apart from this general swelling, many people with PGL feel no ill-effects at all and show no other signs of the infection. Some people with PGL do, however, feel unwell. One of the commonest complaints is of episodes of chronic tiredness. Again, this symptom is variable, affecting some persons far more severely than others. For instance, many patients report feeling very tired and 'drained' of energy for perhaps a week or two, after which they then feel fine for many months. Others report feeling continually affected by fatigue with no intervening periods of relative health and stamina. Those most severely affected may be quite impaired by it so they can no longer function normally at work, at home or recreationally as they used to. The majority of patients with PGL remain as they are and do not get any worse. A minority do, however, experience a further progression of the infection. Why the effects should be so variable is unknown.

3. AIDS-Related Complex (ARC)

Some people infected with HTLV-III will develop a state called ARC. In ARC the immune system has been considerably damaged, but not usually as badly as it is in AIDS patients. As a result of the damage, ARC patients are more susceptible to infection but without showing the tumours or opportunistic infections that would qualify for a diagnosis of AIDS. The numbers of people progressing from ARC to AIDS is higher than the numbers progressing from PGL to AIDS, reflecting the fact that there is a greater degree of damage to the immune system. Common symptoms seen in ARC are listed in Table 1.

Some clinicians prefer not to use the term ARC, and make reference instead to PGL with (i.e. ARC) or without symptoms. However, some patients may have ARC without lymphadenopathy.

In order to fulfil the diagnostic requirements for ARC, only one symptom, one clinical sign and one abnormality arising from laboratory testing is required. As soon as any opportunist infection or tumour associated with a diagnosis of AIDS is discovered (if at all), the diagnosis changes to AIDS.

Table 1: Symptoms and Signs of AIDS-Related Complex (ARC)

SYMPTOMS
severe malaise, lethargy, fatigue
loss of more than 10 per cent bodyweight
more than one month's unexplained diarrhoea
night sweats and/or fevers

SIGNS
oral candida (thrush)
oral leucoplakia
PGL
splenomegaly (enlarged spleen)
eczema/folliculitis

ARC may be a debilitating illness for some people, particularly when waking hours are filled with responding to diarrhoea and sleeping hours are disrupted constantly by fevers and sweats. There is often fatigue and a general feeling of malaise. The social disruption caused by eczema and other conditions can be particularly upsetting. We have often seen patients become chronically depressed and sometimes suicidal in the face of the tremendous disruption caused by ARC.

4. *Acquired Immune Deficiency Syndrome (AIDS)*
From the preceding patient groups, it is currently thought that about 10–15% will go on to develop AIDS within 36 months. AIDS is a highly complex illness potentially involving many infections and tumours (popularly called cancers), although even within the context of AIDS it is difficult to

predict who will and will not develop each of the many illnesses that may arise. The range of infections and tumours commonly seen in people with AIDS is shown in Table 2.

The disorders described in Table 2 are typically seen in patients with other causes of cellular immune deficiencies, for instance those who have received immunosuppressive treatment after major organ transplants (where such treatment is required to reduce the risks of transplant rejection). However, it is clear that which particular illnesses emerge in a patient with AIDS depends to some degree at least on the patient's country of origin, previous history of sexually transmitted diseases, and exposure to different infections before the illness developed. The diagnosis of AIDS requires the presence of an infection or tumour which is extremely rare in those who do not have a severely impaired immune system appearing in a patient for whom no other cause of immune system damage can be found. Although this appears a rather vague definition, in practice it works very well and cases of people being wrongly diagnosed as having AIDS are extremely rare.

There are a number of these infections and tumours which are seen in AIDS patients and these can be most easily classified through the areas of the body in which they appear most often.

1. *Chest infections in AIDS*
The most common infection in AIDS is pneumocystis carinii pneumonia (PCP). This chest infection is seen in about 50% of all initial AIDS diagnoses, and about 60% of all AIDS cases develop PCP at some stage of their illness. Distressingly, PCP is a major cause of death in AIDS, and it tends to appear in those whose immune systems are particularly badly damaged. Early forecasts of survival with PCP were gloomy, but these were probably over-pessimistic: adequate treatment procedures for managing this infection

Table 2: Common Infections and Tumours seen in AIDS in the UK

Agents	Sites of Infection	Common clinical manifestations
PARASITIC		
Pneumocystis carinii	Lungs	Pneumonia
Toxoplasma gondii	Brain	Focal neurological signs
	Lymph nodes, blood	Disseminated infections*
Crytosporidium	Intestine	Diarrhoea
VIRAL		
Herpes simplex (1)	Mouth, genitals, buttocks, hands, brain	Painful ulcerative lesions
		Disseminated infections*
Cytomegalovirus	Lungs	Pneumonia
	Brain	Encephalopathy
	Intestine, bowel	Colitis
	Eye	Retinitis (loss of vision)
	Lymph nodes, liver, blood	Disseminated infections*
BACTERIAL		
Salmonella typhimurium	Intestine	Diarrhoea
	Blood	Septicaemia, fevers
Shigella flexneri	Intestine	Diarrhoea
Mycobacterium tuberculosis	Lung, GI tract	Pneumonia, pleural effusions
Mycobacterium xenopi/kansasii	Lung, GI tract	Disseminated infections*, meningitis, diarrhoea, GI bleeding
FUNGAL		
Candida albicans (2)	Mouth, throat, oesophagus	Oral thrush, pain on swallowing
	Lung, brain	Pneumonia
Cryptococcus neoformans	Brain	Meningitis
	Lungs	Pneumonia
Tinea (3)	Skin	Rash
NEOPLASTIC		
Kaposi's sarcoma	Skin, mouth, anus, gut, respiratory tract	Single, or clusters of, lesions
Lymphoma	Brain, gut	

* Disseminated infections refers to lung, internal organ and/or multiple lymph node involvement.
(1)(2) Herpes and Candida are only diagnostic of AIDS if disseminated.
(3) Tinea is a normal finding and does not indicate that a person has AIDS or is even immunosuppressed.

Adapted from V. Daniels, *AIDS*, Lancaster: MTP Press, 1985

have been developed. The success of management really depends on the speed with which signs of PCP are recognised and treated, as the infection can flare out of control in a matter of days. Many patients currently find that with the greater understanding of treatment alternatives now available, attacks of PCP can be controlled quite quickly and there may be extended periods of remission (free of PCP infection) lasting many months. Signs to look out for in PCP include:

a Shortness of breath during and after periods of exertion.
b Persistent non-productive ('dry') cough.
c Fevers and night sweats.
d Mild chest pain (as in pleurisy).

A number of other chest diseases are also seen in AIDS. The most frequently seen are cytomegalovirus (CMV), a virus infection which often affects other parts of the body, myco-bacterium tuberculosis and mycobacterium xenopi/kansasii, candida albicans, which is a thrush-like infection in the lung giving rise to a pneumonia-like disease, and Kaposi's sarcoma which appears to occur less often with fevers than does PCP.

2. Gastro-intestinal infections in AIDS

The gastro-intestinal region covers the mouth, throat, stomach, intestines and anus. AIDS-related illnesses in these regions are sometimes hard to diagnose, but when they are active they can be overwhelming for the patient. Typical symptoms include diarrhoea and a loss of 10% or more body weight; as these are frequently seen in the context of ARC, the doctor has to perform a thorough series of investigations to reach the correct diagnosis. Other major clinical symptoms include colicky abdominal pains, abdominal distention, anal discomfort or ulceration, and dysphagia (difficulty in swallowing). Of course these symptoms appear in other illnesses. In order to make a diagnosis of AIDS the specific infection responsible has to be identified and it has to be one of those associated with AIDS. Infections which fall into this category include:

a Candida. Candida is very common in AIDS. It is a yeast which is often found in the mouths of healthy people and in the vaginal tract of healthy women, where it can sometimes cause thrush. In AIDS patients it can cause severe problems. Often 'plaques' (large patches) of candida can be seen around the underside of the tongue. These can be quite extensive and can be scraped off easily. Candida can extend down the throat to the stomach, and can cause some mild pain upon swallowing food and drink. This sort of infection is also seen in other situations than AIDS: it can be the result of prolonged treatment with antibiotics, for instance. Such causes need to be excluded. Candidiasis is not diagnostic of AIDS by itself but is a common problem in AIDS patients and ARC patients.

b Cryptosporidiosis. Cryptosporidium is a parasite which produces a short self-limiting illness usually seen in travellers from abroad or people working with cattle. However, in AIDS patients it produces a profuse watery diarrhoea which can be fatal. At present there is no really effective drug to treat it.

c Salmonella and shigella. These bacteria can be a significant problem in people with AIDS, as they have no facility for eliminating them as have those with a normally functioning immune system. These infections produce an enteritis – an inflammation of the intestines – which in itself can usually be managed reasonably successfully, but also a bacteraemia – a presence of the bacteria in the blood – which produces fevers and spreads the disease throughout the body. This requires intravenous antibiotic therapy, without which it may be fatal. These bacteria are found typically in undercooked poultry, so all patients should be warned to take great care in preparing such foods.

d Herpes virus. Genital herpes (due to herpes simplex virus type 2) is a common infection, particularly in very sexually active people. The infection is usually self-limiting – the attacks are short and soon clear up, leaving little or no lasting damage. In AIDS patients it can be more severe and recurrent, producing painful ulceration particularly in the area around the anus. These attacks can now be suppressed using a drug called acyclovir.

e Cytomegalovirus (CMV) infection. CMV infection of the large bowel or colon (colitis) is a common manifestation of AIDS, producing chronic diarrhoea with blood and mucus, pain and abdominal distention, fever and malaise and weight loss. Ulceration of the oesophagus (between the mouth and stomach) can make swallowing food and drink painful. New drugs are now becoming available to treat this illness.

f Kaposi's sarcoma (KS). KS is a cancer of the skin but may occur in many other parts of the body, including the membranes lining the lungs, the liver, bone, etc. In the majority of cases such lesions produce few if any symptoms. However, occasionally they will cause severe pneumonia, or gastro-intestinal problems such as diarrhoea or bleeding.

3. Skin disorders in AIDS

There are three main categories of skin disorders in the context of AIDS: Kaposi's sarcoma (KS), skin infections following from the effects of immune suppression, both of which are discussed below, and non-specific disorders such as seborrhoeic dermatitis and eczema.

a Kaposi's sarcoma. About 25% of all people with AIDS are first diagnosed with the skin tumour KS, and another 10% will suffer this disorder after initially being diagnosed with an opportunist infection. For reasons unknown, the appearance of KS seems to depend largely on the risk group of the patient. For example, while about 45% of male homosexual AIDS patients develop KS, it is very rare for haemophiliacs to do so. This peculiarity may be due to the presence of various 'co-factors', that is, the higher prevalence of other infections in homosexual populations, CMV in particular. It has also been suggested that the use of stimulant drugs such as amyl nitrites may play a part. The question remains unresolved at the moment.

KS can occur anywhere on the skin or the mucous membranes lining the body cavities and may appear as a small pink raised bump or a dark purple patch or bump of about 1cm diameter. They may increase in size or shrink and even disappear. They are painless, do not blanch on pressure and do not itch. People at risk understandably worry greatly about any new skin lesion, and this anxiety in itself may make certain skin rashes worse. It is important to be able to recognise these lesions, and reassure patients when they have no cause for concern.

Patients with KS alone have the best prognosis in all studies conducted so far. The development and course of AIDS with KS is directly related to the degree of immunosuppression the person is suffering, so it is important that they avoid any activities or involvements that may further lower their immunity (see Chapter 9).

The severity of Kaposi's sarcoma varies greatly, and may be dependent on the degree of immunosuppression present. The majority of patients have no symptoms and have only a few lesions requiring no therapy, although if these lesions occur on the face and hands they can be very distressing and the use of make-up or of local radiotherapy to decrease their size may be recommended. Occasionally severe widespread lesions require drug therapy to control them.

b Skin infections. Other skin conditions appearing in the context of AIDS include herpes simplex, which was discussed earlier, molluscum contagiosum – a viral infection producing pearly raised spots, usually on the face or body, fungal rashes such as tinea, and non-specific skin disorders such as eczema and folliculitis, both of which are relatively easily treated. These skin problems also, of course, appear often in people who do not have AIDS.

4. Central Nervous System (CNS) disorders in AIDS
This group of disorders in AIDS refers to damage in the brain and spinal cord.

The CNS is susceptible to both opportunist infections and tumours. The most common infection is cryptococcal meningitis, a fungal condition that causes headaches, fevers, difficulties in co-ordination and walking, visual problems, epileptic-type fits and memory disturbances. Toxoplasmosis can cause abscesses in the brain, producing focal neurological problems such as paralysis of the limbs, speech problems, weakness of the face or epileptic fits.

A proportion of people with AIDS show evidence of 'AIDS encephalopathy' – a progressive 'shrinking' of the brain resulting, in very severe cases, in the sorts of symptoms seen in dementia in the elderly. The patient may therefore demonstrate a loss of memory, poor orientation (they don't know where they are, the date, have problems recognising family and friends), speech difficulties, loss of bodily control (including co-ordination in walking), poor concentration and easy distractability and, in more severe cases, changes in personality. Epileptic fits may also appear in this context. This is a particularly distressing condition as it so profoundly affects the patient's relationship with lover, spouse and family. It is thought that the infection responsible for this deterioration may be HTLV-III itself. In some cases, CMV or cryptococcus may be responsible and these are treatable, whereas encephalopathy due to HTLV-III is not, as yet. It must be stressed that the majority of AIDS patients do not show this severe pattern of central nervous system damage.

It still remains a puzzle as to why some people infected with the virus go on to develop AIDS while others do not. There are a number of probable reasons. People who go on to get AIDS probably have more 'co-factors', other infections, particularly sexually transmitted infections. These may help the virus to produce AIDS. General health may possibly also be a factor. The better state the immune system is in in the first place, the better the chance of resisting the infection. It may also be that there is a certain amount of variation in the way in which different people's immune systems respond to the virus. Some may produce a certain amount of effective neutralising antibody, for instance, though this has not been conclusively shown as yet. It may also be that there are different strains of the virus with different abilities to cause AIDS, although this is purely conjecture.

It is important to discover why some people get AIDS rapidly after infection with HTLV-III and some do not. In finding an answer it may be possible to find new ways of treating AIDS itself.

Chapter Five

POSSIBLE ORIGINS

From time to time a new disease sweeps the word. In the fourteenth century bubonic plague, the Black Death, killed a quarter to a third of the populations of China, India and Europe. It probably started in Central Asia, where the bacterium which causes the disease was present in a reservoir of small mammals. Floods, earthquakes or other natural disasters in that area may have caused the migration of these infected animals out of the small geographical area where they lived. At some point they passed the disease on to people.

Once the plague was in the human population it moved down through China, along the trade routes from China to India, from there to the Middle East and then, on the trading ships that carried silk and spices, to the great trading ports of Italy. Once it had a foothold in Europe it spread throughout the continent, finally reaching England from France, the Low Countries and Scandinavia. The moment was perfect for the spread. The trade routes were busier than ever before, since political stability in the areas through which they passed had brought a new confidence to the merchants with rising demands for the products of the East that brought new profits.

The spread of bubonic plague is an interesting example of two ways in which new diseases emerge. The first is the spread of a disease which has been confined to a small area by means of improved travel or movements of population: it has been argued that the ships of Christopher Columbus brought back syphilis from the New World to the Old World. Secondly, a disease present in animals may spread to man. In 1967 laboratory workers in Marburg, West Germany, were infected by a virus that they caught from a batch of Ugandan vervet monkeys. This was a new disease never before seen in the West, although further outbreaks of Marburg virus have been recognised in Africa. Bubonic plague originated in animals and was spread not only from person to person but also by fleas from infected rats.

A third way in which new diseases start is by mutation, particularly of viruses. Periodic influenza epidemics are caused by a mutated virus. The influenza virus changes from time to time so that people who have built up immunity to the old strains of the virus no longer have that immunity and, from time to time, a great influenza pandemic sweeps the world: the influenza epidemic of the second decade of the twentieth century killed more people than the First World War. HTLV-III is a virus which seems to mutate particularly rapidly.

The most likely source of HTLV-III is Africa. There is evidence that HTLV-III, or a very closely related virus which might have mutated into HTLV-III, has been present in Africa for at least ten to fifteen years, and possibly longer. In the West there is at present no evidence for infection earlier than seven or eight years ago, despite the wider availability than in Africa of stored blood samples from the past. This suggests that HTLV-III was present in Africa before it appeared in the West. However, the further we go back into the stored blood samples of Africa, the fewer the people that seem to have been infected with such a virus. This would suggest that, in most of Africa, the virus is a new one.

There are two possible explanations of this. Firstly, it may be that the virus was always present in some small, geographically isolated part of Africa, among people with few contacts with the outside world. With the increasing shift from the countryside to the towns in the sixties and seventies, and the increasing opening-up of Africa by better roads, the virus might have spread out of its base. Although this is an appealing idea, it would seem that because of the high infant mortality from HTLV-III infection it would be more likely to have wiped out such an isolated group of people. One way round this is to argue that a closely-related virus may have been present in such a tribe, which at some point over the last thirty years has mutated to produce HTLV-III.

The other suggestion, which seems more plausible, is that HTLV-III was originally an animal virus. What makes this such an intriguing idea is that a number of similar viruses are known in animals. One of the closest relatives of HTLV-III is an Icelandic sheep virus, the Visna virus, although it seems unlikely that Icelandic sheep could have provided the source of HTLV-III, and that virus does not transfer to man. Other viruses similar to HTLV-III include a cattle retrovirus, bovine leukaemia virus, and a virus of pigs. Some African tribes drink the blood of their cattle, so a cattle virus has some attractions. There are many other animal retroviruses which are similar to HTLV-III.

The virus which is most likely as a starting point is STLV-III, Simian T-cell lymphotropic virus, which has caused a number of outbreaks of an AIDS-like illness in monkeys in North American zoos. It infects both the macacque monkey and the green monkey. The virus is very similar genetically to HTLV-III. Monkeys are our nearest evolutionary relatives and are able to pass on a number of diseases to humans. The blood of some Africans infected with HTLV-III reacts with STLV-III, suggesting that the viruses are very similar to one another. There is also evidence that some Africans, in particular West Africans, may be infected with STLV-III itself, or a virus very close to it. They show no symptoms from their infection. The process can also work the other way: it is possible artificially to infect monkeys with HTLV-III itself.

The blood of American HTLV-III infected subjects is less likely to react with STLV-III virus than African blood, suggesting that the virus they have has mutated further, so that it is much more different from STLV-III than African HTLV-III.

Overall, the best suggestion as to the origins of HTLV-III is this. HTLV-III was originally a monkey virus, either STLV-III or a very similar virus. Some monkeys seem rather resistant to possible ill-effects from STLV-III, so it could have been present in monkeys for many years. The virus spread to people in some way. Studies of another monkey virus which can infect man, monkey pox, have shown a number of intriguing facts. Monkeys are often hunted for food in Africa. It may be that a hunting accident of some sort, or an accident in preparation for cooking, brought people into contact with infected blood. Once caught, monkeys are often kept in huts for some time before they are eaten. Dead monkeys are sometimes used as toys by African children.

Once the virus entered the human population it probably mutated rapidly, as it is doing now. The movement of people from rural areas to the cities, and the greater general mobility of the population of Africa, would mean that such a virus would spread far more readily now than at any previous time in the history of Africa. With the shift in population, particularly young single men, to the towns came a greater use of prostitutes than previously, and this would have provided a ready mechanism for spread.

If this was the case, how could the virus have reached the West? There are several possibilities. The most likely route is cheap air travel, which allowed many Americans to travel to Central Africa in the seventies. In the process a number of them had sex with local people, both heterosexual and homosexual sex. From that point the virus could easily have gained a foothold in America. There is also the possibility that interchanges of professional people between Haiti and Central Africa in the sixties and seventies may have provided a route, though that seems less likely. Many American gay men holidayed in Haiti and there was a ready availability of male prostitutes in that very poor country.

Haitian immigrants were at one time classified as a separate risk group for AIDS. It is now recognised that their relatively high rate of HTLV-III infection reflects the usual routes of transmission. Because of the extreme poverty of Haiti, some otherwise heterosexual Haitian men were prepared to engage in homosexual prostitution and unwilling to admit their activities to early researchers. Export of HTLV-III to Haiti from America seems likely to have been the main factor in the high rates of infection seen in immigrants from that country.

One notion that is clearly not true is the idea that HTLV-III was imported somehow with the slave trade. There is no evidence that American or Caribbean black people had HTLV-III infections before the 1970s. The virus probably appeared in Africa long after the slave trade ended.

People generally think of diseases as always being the same, and think that the appearance of a new disease is something odd. It is in fact an almost commonplace event. New diseases are constantly being identified (Legionnaires' disease, for instance) which were previously not recognised, or are appearing for the first time, in the West at least (including Lassa fever and Marburg virus disease). Sometimes new diseases seem to appear from nowhere and disappear as suddenly as did encephalitis lethargica in the early part of this century.

.Other geographically isolated areas with similar characteristics to Central Africa have been suggested as the most likely starting point for the current HTLV-III epidemic. South America, particularly the Amazon basin, an area cut off from the outside world and with a high monkey population which might form a reservoir for an animal virus, has been favoured by some researchers. There is no convincing evidence at present that either the monkey population or the local tribesmen of these areas are in fact infected with HTLV-III or something like it. Moreover, it is hard to see how the virus could have travelled to Africa from these areas and how it could have got there before it got to North America, which has much stronger links with South America in terms of trade and tourism.

It will probably never be possible to be certain, but the current evidence in favour of an African origin is strong. Recently two new viruses, LAV-2 and HTLV-IV have been reported in Central Africans. They may be the same virus and they appear to be intermediate between HTLV-III and STLV-III strengthening the case for an African origin. What the evidence does show clearly is that ordinary, commonplace, biological mechanisms are quite adequate to explain the appearance of HTLV-III. There is no need to cast around for ideas that the virus was built in a laboratory or the result of nuclear testing. New diseases have been appearing in the West on a regular basis since long before there were nuclear bombs or laboratories.

One more chilling fact also comes out of the story. HTLV-III is not the first new virus we have seen. There is every reason to suppose that it will not be the last.

Chapter Six

HOW DOES HTLV-III SPREAD?

The first thing to establish is how HTLV-III does not spread. A glance at the popular press could leave anyone with the feeling that the virus is extremely infectious and that people who have it are a grave threat to others. Nothing could be further from the truth. The newspapers carry stories of people being barred from bars and clubs because they are homosexual, of court cases in which HTLV-III infected prisoners are accompanied by prison officers in protective suits, of workmates shunning AIDS sufferers and putting them in separate offices. All this is simply hysteria.

HTLV-III is a virus which is spread in three ways, through blood, through sex and from mother to child in the womb, at birth or through breast-milk. It is not spread through the air, like cold and influenza viruses, it is not spread by touching someone, it cannot be caught from cups or cutlery. You could be marooned in a lifeboat with fifty AIDS sufferers for a month and suffer nothing worse than seasickness. There is no risk in sharing cutlery, crockery and cups because there is very little virus in saliva and even if there were any in saliva on the rim of a cup, it would not be enough to infect anyone. In any case, ordinary washing-up destroys the virus.

Similarly the lavatory, the focus of many people's fears of contagion, conveys no risk. You cannot catch HTLV-III from a lavatory seat, nor can you catch it from baths or washbasins. No special hygiene precautions are necessary. It is also not possible to catch it from towels, although common sense dictates that a towel that is heavily contaminated with blood should not be shared with anyone.

Most sets of guidelines on the control of infection suggest that toothbrushes and wet-shave razors should not be shared with anyone else. Many people bleed from their gums when they brush their teeth and the toothbrush may become contaminated with blood; many people cut themselves when they are shaving. There is no evidence that anyone has ever caught the virus in either of these ways, but keeping your own toothbrush and razor – or switching to an electric razor – are hardly onerous measures.

The only other potential area of difficulty is if someone with HTLV-III infection sustains a cut while, say, preparing a meal and then bleeds all over the salad and the work surfaces. What should be done? Well, the first thing is to stop the bleeding and put a plaster on the cut. The next thing is to throw away the salad, because no one likes eating blood-stained lettuce. After that all that is necessary is to mop up the blood with a paper towel or something similar, and then flush the paper down the lavatory. Someone else mopping it up should wear ordinary household gloves. For extra safety, washing down surfaces in one part ordinary bleach to ten parts water will destroy any virus lurking in blood that may have been missed.

These are common-sense actions. In practice, providing your skin is intact, and you do not have eczema or a recent cut or other damage, there is no real risk of catching the virus: it is simply incapable of penetrating intact skin. Of course, if anyone bleeds on you, you will wash the blood off with soap and water, which nicely kills the virus in the process.

The clothes of someone with HTLV-III infection can be washed in the normal way with those of the rest of the family if necessary. If they are heavily stained with blood or other body fluids they can be washed on a hot temperature on their own, but that is something people would normally do. No one ever caught HTLV-III from a shirt, anyway. No one should be worried about using commercial launderettes: they are quite safe.

Kissing and cuddling is an issue that many HTLV-III infected people suffer agonies about. They are afraid that they will pass on the virus to their mothers and fathers, sons and daughters or nephews and nieces in this way. They can be completely reassured. The virus cannot be passed on by this kind of contact, nor can it be passed on by shaking hands or sitting next to someone on the bus. As a matter of fact, it is reassuring to know that no one anywhere in the world has ever caught HTLV-III through normal everyday social contacts or through domestic items such as toothbrushes and razors.

The virus can be found in a number of body fluids. The most important of these are blood, semen and vaginal and cervical secretions.

BLOOD

There is no doubt that the virus can be passed on through blood. Both in Europe and the United States there have been cases of people having blood transfusions acquiring HTLV-III from infected donations. With the introduction of screening of all blood donations, and strong efforts to dissuade those in high-risk groups from giving blood, this is no longer likely to be a source of infection.

Although the virus is found in blood there is little risk to the average person from someone infected with the virus who happens to be bleeding. The blood or virus from the blood would actually have to enter the body of a person for the infection to be passed on. Since neither blood nor virus can penetrate intact skin this is very unlikely. In theory, someone infected with the virus might bleed into a cut on someone's skin and infect them in that way: in practice, the cut would have to be a very new one, since the processes which protect cuts against infection occur very rapidly after injury. In any case, how many people would let someone else bleed into their cut? There has never been a case in which anyone has caught the virus in this way and it is not something that the average person in the street should be at all worried about.

Some very reassuring information comes from health workers. Doctors, nurses and other health staff have far more direct contact with blood and other body fluids than any member of the general public is likely to have. Until 1983 AIDS was not known to be infectious. Health staff took no special precautions whatsoever with patients. Today there may be a million people in the US infected with the virus, most of whom are unaware of the fact. Many of these are being operated on, having injections and generally being looked after with no special precautions, simply because no one knows that they are infected. Despite all this, there has never been a case of AIDS in a health professional as a result of their work.

One health professional, a British nurse, and probably two others in the United States have been infected with HTLV-III in the course of their duties. In each case the method of infection was a needle-stick injury, in which a professional who is taking blood from an infected patient suffers a self-inflicted puncture. At the same time there have been well over 650 needle-stick accidents reported involving infected patients in which no infection occurred in the health professional. This fact underlines the low infectivity of this virus. Needle-stick injuries do not happen to the average man or woman. If doctors and nurses are not catching HTLV-III through the close contact they have with patients, then the man in the street has nothing to fear from casual everyday contact.

SEMEN

Many people infected with HTLV-III have virus in their semen and can infect other people by ejaculating into the vagina or rectum. This seems to be the main route for infection in vaginal intercourse. There has recently been a case in Australia where a number of women had artificial insemination by donor with infected semen and became infected with HTLV-III. To prevent this sort of thing happening again all semen donors are screened to ensure that they are free of HTLV-III. High-risk donors are asked not to donate semen in the same way as they are asked not to give blood. The only problem here is that a number of lesbian women would like to have semen donations from gay men, which does present some risk. For the recipient with no such preferences there should be no risk.

Before ejaculation men tend to produce a pre-ejaculatory secretion. It is not known whether or not this contains the virus, but at the moment it is probably sensible to assume that it does: infection may possibly occur during intercourse even without ejaculation if this is so.

VAGINAL AND CERVICAL SECRETIONS

Virus has recently been isolated from vaginal and cervical secretions and it is probable that this is the way in which women can infect men through vaginal intercourse.

73

SALIVA

Nothing has worried ordinary people so much as the finding of virus in the saliva of a proportion of infected people, but this is not something which causes any great concern for clinicians working in the field. By no means all people who are infected have virus in their saliva, and those who do are very unlikely to be infectious to other people through their saliva.

Firstly, any virus present in saliva is likely to be very dilute and there will be little of it. Secondly, transmission by cups, cutlery and other things that saliva gets on to is impossible. The amount of saliva on, say, a cup, is far too small to cause any problems and is got rid of in ordinary washing-up. There is not a shadow of a doubt that you simply cannot catch HTLV-III in this way. In some bars in America it is now almost impossible to get a glass to drink beer out of: all beer is drunk from the bottle to avoid HTLV-III. This is complete nonsense. What has led to the confusion is the distinction between being able to culture the virus from saliva in the highly artificial environment of the laboratory and saliva's actually being an infection risk in the ordinary everyday world.

For this reason, kissing is not likely to be a risk, whether kissing someone on the cheek or on the lips. Very little saliva is transferred in this way and, in the case of the cheek, it is going on to skin. Deep kissing, in which the tongue is put into someone's mouth and large amounts of saliva are exchanged, is a theoretical risk, but the chances of anyone becoming infected in this way are remote. Certainly no one has ever been known to have been infected by HTLV-III from saliva.

BREAST MILK

The breast milk of women infected with HTLV-III often has the virus in it, even if all cellular material is taken out. Women who are infected or whose sexual partners are in high-risk groups should never breast feed, nor should they donate milk to milk banks.

OTHER BODY FLUIDS

The virus has also been found in tears and, more recently, in urine. It is not necessary to take the idea of infection through these routes seriously. Like saliva there is little virus and it is enormously dilute.

The virus has not been found in faeces as yet, nor has it been found in sweat. No body fluids other than blood or semen are likely to cause any problem.

In fact we know a great deal about the transmission of HTLV-III from the families of people who are infected. One obvious case is those families who have children who are haemophiliacs.

Virtually all haemophiliacs are male. Because haemophilia is passed on by women, who rarely suffer from haemophilia, the parents are usually not haemophiliacs themselves. The sisters of haemophiliacs are similarly not haemophiliac and only 50% of a haemophiliac's brothers will be affected. The typical family of a haemophiliac, then, consists of one child with haemophilia, and parents and brothers and sisters who are not haemophiliac. We know a great deal about these families.

Of all the families with haemophiliac children infected with HTLV-III that have been studied, in no case have non-haemophiliac members of the family been infected with

HTLV-III. This is in spite of the fact that the parents have to handle the body fluids of the child in the way that most parents have to. They cuddle the child, they kiss him, they are in close everyday contact with him. Similarly, the brothers and sisters are never infected either, despite playing with the child and being in close and often fairly unhygienic contact with him. If this sort of contact does not pass on the virus we can be pretty sure that ordinary everyday contact will never pass it on.

Similar studies in Africa of children infected with HTLV-III have shown that the brothers and sisters of those children are rarely infected, and where they are they caught the virus in the same way, i.e., from the mother in the womb or from breast-feeding. Simple everyday contact does not pass on HTLV-III.

There are two main ways in which HTLV-III is passed on, sexually and through blood. It is worth looking at each of these in detail and considering ways in which they can be avoided.

SEXUAL TRANSMISSION

There are very few things which homosexual men do that heterosexuals do not do also. Many homosexual men also have sex with women. Therefore there is little point in making a distinction between homosexuals and heterosexuals as far as sexual practices go. The main sexual risks seem to be the following:

Anal Intercourse
HTLV-III spreads readily in anal intercourse. When someone has anal sex there is often damage to the rectum and anus, which leads to bleeding. Often neither partner is aware

of this happening. Blood can come into contact with the delicate membrane covering the penis and there is often damage to the penis itself. All this means that HTLV-III can be passed on from the person receiving the penis to the person inserting it. But the process also works the other way.

The person inserting the penis is likely to ejaculate or to produce pre-ejaculatory secretion. If he is infected with HTLV-III he can pass this on to his partner either because semen gets into tears in the anus or rectum or by directly infecting the lining of the rectum.

One way to cut down the risk is to use a condom. HTLV-III does not pass across a condom. However, the trouble with condoms is that they can break, and they can break particularly often in anal intercourse. They can also slip off. This is because the muscles around the anus go into spasm and exert a particularly high mechanical strain on the condom, far more than in vaginal intercourse. Some work on London prostitutes carried out at St Mary's Hospital showed that some of the female prostitutes who were having anal intercourse using condoms with their clients reported up to a 50% failure rate. This can probably be reduced by using a lubricant cream, but even so the rate of failure is unacceptably high.

It seems safest for people to avoid anal intercourse totally, since it is something which is difficult to make safe. However, if they cannot do this they should use a condom. Preferably they should use one of the condoms now becoming available which are specially designed for anal intercourse. They are stronger and in theory should be subject to less breakages, although at the moment we do not know how safe they will actually be. Similarly they could still slip. They should always be used with a water-based lubricant.

Inserting objects or fingers into the anus should also be avoided, since this increases the risk of damage to the rectum and there is often a good deal of bleeding.

Vaginal intercourse
Vaginal intercourse is also a way in which HTLV-III can be transmitted. Whether there needs to be a small amount of damage to the vagina or whether the virus directly infects the intact vagina is of mainly theoretical interest. Either way it is extremely common or there would not be so many Africans with the virus or so many female sexual partners of infected men with the virus in the West.

Again, the only totally safe way to deal with the problem is to avoid vaginal intercourse. However, condoms probably provide a greater degree of protection in vaginal intercourse, for the simple reason that they do not break or slip as often. Every woman who has a partner who is infected or who may be in a high-risk group should use condoms all the time if they intend to continue with vaginal intercourse. They should also use a back-up method of contraception to avoid pregnancy.

If a woman who is infected with HTLV-III becomes pregnant there is a very strong – perhaps 50–50 – chance that the baby will also be infected. If the baby is infected it is very likely to develop AIDS, again there is perhaps a 50% chance. This is because the baby's immune system is so under-developed. At the same time the mother herself is likely to be at grave risk. During pregnancy the immune system is impaired and the woman is at much greater risk of getting AIDS if she is infected. An infected woman who does not develop AIDS during one pregnancy may do so during a subsequent pregnancy. Where the father is infected and the mother is not there is always the risk that the ejaculation which makes her pregnant will also be the one which makes her infected. The risks are just not worth taking.

Therefore if a woman is using condoms she should also take other steps to make doubly sure she will not get pregnant. The pill is probably a good method; so is the cap. Indeed the cap may have other advantages. It protects the cervix, and this may be one of the sites where HTLV-III is likely to infect a woman. Unfortunately we do not know if this is the only site of infection of the vagina or whether the rest of the vaginal barrel can also be infected. At the moment it seems safest to assume that the whole vagina is susceptible to infection so that a cap alone is probably not sufficient protection by itself. However, a condom plus cap plus spermicide may well be a good combination both to prevent pregnancy and to avoid infection.

There is good reason to suggest that every man and woman who is having casual sex should insist on the use of a condom. This is not just to protect against HTLV-III. The condom offers some degree of protection against a whole range of sexually transmitted disease from syphilis to herpes. It also protects the cervix against wart virus, as does the cap. Wart virus may well be responsible for the recent alarming increase in cancer of the cervix in young sexually active women.

Oral sex

No one knows just how risky oral sex is. There are two issues which are difficult to sort out. The first involves the man ejaculating into the mouth of his partner or producing a pre-ejaculatory secretion. This may well be infected with virus. On the other hand there have been no cases in which the virus has definitely been passed on in this way. Attempts to infect monkeys through their mouths by putting in live virus have failed (they can be readily infected anally or vaginally). Gay men who only engage in oral sex do not seem to be infected with the virus. On the other hand if someone has cuts or ulcers in their mouths it is possible that they may be infected with the virus through oral sex.

The second issue concerns the virus in saliva or from blood from cuts or damage in the mouth. This can get either on to the penis or the vagina. Saliva has already been discussed earlier and the risks from this source appear to be small.

There is one other issue worth considering. While HTLV-III may or may not be passed on in oral sex, other sexually transmitted diseases most certainly can be. In someone already infected with HTLV-III, catching these can worsen one's outlook a good deal.

Overall, the best advice seems to be to avoid oral sex at least until we know more. If someone is going to engage in oral sex ejaculation into the mouth is to be totally avoided.

One final issue in oral sex is oral–anal contact. This is always a very risky business and should be completely avoided. There is no way it can be made safe and we have always told our patients not to do it unless they can get a condom on their tongue!

What is safe sexually
Some things can be done with impunity. Mutual masturbation presents essentially no risk. Intact skin is coming into contact with the penis or vagina and for that reason there should be no infection. Of course it would be different if someone had cuts or sores on their hands, but who would engage in mutual masturbation with cuts and sores on their hands?

Body-rubbing (rubbing the penis or clitoris against the partner's body) should also present no risks unless there is obvious damage to the skin.

In fact if people were to stick only to these two sexual activities they could sleep with as many people as they wanted and be at virtually no risk. Unfortunately these practices do not have the attractions of anal or vaginal intercourse for most people. They can be made interesting and fun but they need imagination and ingenuity to make them exciting.

For most people trying to make their sex lives safer it is much easier to sort things out with a single partner than with multiple partners. It is easier to agree with someone you know well exactly what you will and will not do. And, of course, in a stable monogamous relationship where both partners are free from HTLV-III there is no risk of catching the virus.

TRANSMISSION THROUGH BLOOD

Transmission through blood is not a real risk for most people. The chances of getting HTLV-III through a blood transfusion are now extremely remote and not worth worrying about. Even for haemophiliacs the heat-treatment of Factor VIII and blood screening should protect them.

Intravenous drug abusers are a group particularly at risk through sharing syringes with others. They need to acquire a clean syringe of their own and not to share it with others.

Otherwise, anyone who does not habitually engage in blood-brotherhood rites should be pretty safe.

OTHER ISSUES

There are certain steps which people who are infected with this virus should take to protect themselves and others:

- They should not give blood, or donate organs or semen.
- They should not be tattooed, or have their ears pierced or have acupuncture. With good sterile practices none of these things should be a risk but good sterile practices are not always carried out by 'back-street' operators.
- They should lead normal lives and ignore most of the things which are written in newspapers.
- They should inform their doctor and dentist that they are infected. However, the best advice is that if you think your doctor or dentist will not be discreet and sympathetic, change them.

81

If a doctor or dentist knows that someone is infected they may be able to pick up any health problems the patient has early in the day, and thus treat the patient more rapidly and effectively.

In summary, if nothing else people should appreciate that this is a sexually transmitted disease. It *can* be passed on through blood but the risks of this happening to the average person in the street are so small as not to be worth worrying about. Other than by these two routes – sexually and through blood – no one in the general population is at risk of catching HTLV-III.

Chapter Seven

THE RISK GROUPS I:
Homosexual Men

Homosexuality has been present in all cultures and at all times in history, at least as far as we know. References to homosexuality go back as far as Babylon. It is expressly condemned in the Bible, it was fashionable in ancient Athens, many of the great Roman poets and writers were homosexual, or at least bisexual. At most times and in most cultures it has been at least viewed as an inferior form of sexuality and often it has been savagely persecuted. The example of homosexuality in England is typical.

It is clear that homosexuality existed in the Middle Ages. Anal intercourse between men was an ecclesiastical offence, that is, it came under the jurisdiction of the church. The penalty was to be burnt at the stake, although it seems not to have been very commonly applied. It was only in 1553 that Henry VIII transferred the offence to the civil courts, when the penalty became hanging. In contrast, the last burning of a homosexual at the stake in France was as late as 1772.

Despite these savage penalties homosexual activities continued. Edward II, King of England, was homosexual. He was deposed and murdered by having a red-hot poker inserted into his rectum through a drinking horn. The method was intended to get rid of him without too many marks showing, but there seems little doubt that his murderers thought it a just punishment for his sexuality.

The Elizabethan era was one of further repression, but a number of the men who contributed to the great age of English literature seem to have been homosexual. The playwright Christopher Marlowe, author of *Doctor Faustus* and also of a play about Edward II, was murdered in a homosexual brawl in Deptford (although the possibility that the occasion provided an opportunity to get rid of him for political reasons cannot be discounted).

Although the death penalty was enforceable for anal intercourse it seems to have been used rarely; the usual punishment for homosexual anal sex in the seventeenth and eighteenth centuries was to be put in the pillory. There the unfortunate man stood, his head and hands through the wooden restraint, quite unable to defend himself. It was not unusual for people in the pillory to be badly injured or even killed by the mob who, if they were not sympathetic to the offence, would stone the offender. Although the last man in England to be hanged for homosexual intercourse was Captain Robert James at the astonishingly late date of 1772, by the eighteenth century behaviour was a little more relaxed. The first gay clubs opened in London, and a number of prominent figures in political and social life were homosexual, or at least presumed to be so, but no action was taken to prosecute them.

The nineteenth century brought the strangely hypocritical attitude associated with the Victorians, although it preceded Queen Victoria's ascent to the throne. The Victorians were prudes in the drawing-room but libertines in the bedroom. Every night thousands of prostitutes thronged the streets of London. The more expensive courtesans were frequented by the great men of the age and many grew rich, sometimes even marrying into the aristocracy. There was an enormous market for pornography, particularly sado-masochism. A huge gap existed between what was considered acceptable for men and for women. Upper-class men kept their wives under close scrutiny, and the life of these women was restricted by social conventions tighter than the corsets they wore. At the same time, the men consorted on a large scale with prostitutes, partly because of the late age of marriage for men and partly because prostitutes offered social and sexual freedoms that could not be exercised at home.

Many upper-class men who would never have dreamed of having sex with a man had strong emotional relationships with other men. Such relationships were the subject of much social approval; the biblical story of David and Jonathan was much quoted and loved. Even so, with hindsight, it seems likely that many such friendships went rather further emotionally than the participants admitted, even to themselves. At the same time, homosexual activity was easier than it had been before. In particular there was a large market for paid sex. Male prostitutes, although fewer than female prostitutes, were easy to come by. There were a number of homosexual brothels in London, associated with several scandals in the nineteenth century involving prominent public figures. The Victorians would tolerate a great deal providing it was done in secret and there was no publicity. It was really the existence of homosexual prostitutes that offended many of the more influential Members of Parliament. As they walked from their clubs to the House they could hardly fail to notice the numbers of young men openly soliciting in the streets and the scandals over homosexual brothels were something they could hardly ignore.

It was largely these factors which influenced the drafting of the Criminal Law Amendment Act of 1885. The law had already been changed in 1861, when anal intercourse ceased to be a capital offence and a maximum sentence of life imprisonment had been substituted, but the 1885 Act introduced a new element. Before that time anal intercourse had been the offence, but the new law outlawed all homosexual acts, including oral sex, between men. It is doubtful whether those who drafted the Bill intended this to happen (the change was the result of a section mainly aimed at controlling the exploitation of women), but the effect of the Criminal Law Amendment Act was dramatically to widen the grounds on which homosexual men could be prosecuted.

An odd sidelight on attitudes to homosexuality is cast up by the Criminal Law Amendment Act. Although male homosexuals were to be strongly punished, lesbians were excluded from the Act. The then Prime Minister, Palmerston, claimed that the reason for the exclusion was that no one had the courage to tell Queen Victoria that lesbianism existed. The truth of the matter seems to be that examples of states directly persecuting lesbians are extremely rare. As far as the criminal law goes at least, female homosexuality has never faced the systematic legal persecution that male homosexuality has, although social persecution has been common. Perhaps this is because most laws have been made by men who find lesbianism less offensive than male homosexuality. Indeed, it forms such a common theme in pornography that it seems likely that many men find it at least mildly titillating.

The first move towards the legalisation of homosexuality came with the Wolfenden Report in 1957. The Government committee took the view that what people did in bed together was not an affair for the state. Even so, it took until 1967 for the law to change to legalise homosexuality in England and Wales and stringent conditions were imposed. The age of consent was set at 21, rather than the 16 years for heterosexuals. The armed forces and merchant seamen were excluded. The law specifies homosexual acts between consenting adults in private. The 'in private' means that no more than two persons should be present, so that group sex is illegal for homosexuals but not for heterosexuals. Curiously, anal intercourse between consenting heterosexuals remains an offence.

It is sometimes said that the persecution of homosexuals is a Judaeo–Christian affair, based on the attitudes of the Bible. This is simply untrue. Cultures as far apart as ancient China, India and the Incas of Peru have persecuted homosexuals, often with far more ferocity than the countries of the Western hemisphere.

The most difficult question of all to answer is why governments have so systematically persecuted homosexuals. Undoubtedly the laws they have enforced have often reflected public attitudes. There are signs that these attitudes are changing, but rather more slowly than the laws. Why are people antagonistic to homosexuals? Most of the answers put forward have been unsatisfactory.

Many people when asked why they dislike homosexuals express views in terms of some authority or other: the Bible is a favourite authority. But the Bible contains all kinds of laws concerning sexual, hygiene and dietary practices that few Christians would dream of following these days. Few people would advocate, for instance, that a woman raped within the boundaries of a city should be stoned to death. So why should the strictures on homosexuality command such widespread support?

Some psychoanalysts have put forward the view that many men have unconscious homosexual desires and that persecuting homosexuals is a way of fighting these desires. There really is no evidence at all for this suggestion – no one would suggest that racial prejudice is the result of white people having a secret desire to be black – yet this rather silly idea has gained considerable currency. It is glib, superficially plausible, and rubbish.

Perhaps the analogy between racial prejudice and homosexuality is much closer than it first appears. People have always persecuted those who are different from themselves. Black people are an easy target in most white countries because they are so easy to recognise. Perhaps looking down on others raises a person's self-esteem. Also, people form social groups which define their own identity by contrast to those who are not in 'our gang': maybe prejudice forms a sort of social cement. Class prejudice, racial prejudice, prejudice against other firms competing in your firm's markets, even the mistrust of nations by other nations, may simply be a result of the way people get on together. The more obviously different a group is, the more likely its members are to be persecuted.

Once a group is the subject of persecution, all sorts of myths arise about that group. In the nineteenth century many physicians seriously believed that the penises of black men were much larger than those of white men (in fact there is no difference whatsoever). In Nazi Germany many people believed the Jews were part of an international world conspiracy. Today many people believe that homosexual men are child molesters and deviants. Over the years the target of prejudice changes, but its nature does not.

The search for a cause of homosexuality has not helped in reducing prejudice. Some men prefer women, some prefer men and some are attracted to both. There clearly has to be a reason why this is the case. If we understood why people's preferences are as they are we would know a lot more about human sexuality. Unfortunately, much of the research into the causes of homosexuality has been distorted by a combination of people's prejudices about what homosexuals are like and by mistaken views of what they do. As a simple example, most researchers have taken the view that homosexuals are quite separate from heterosexuals: in fact, as will be discussed later, many men vary in their sexual orientation throughout their lives. This makes it difficult to justify some fixed physical or biochemical cause for homosexuality. Similarly, few theories take account of the fact that many men are attracted to both men and women, again undermining any theory which sees homosexuality as a result of some failure of normal development.

The earliest theories of the origins of homosexuality were in terms of body build. Homosexuals were thought to be more slight, more feminine in their build. These ideas found some support from studies of homosexuals in mental hospitals and other institutions. It does not seem to have occurred to the researchers that in any group which is being systematically persecuted the most physically weak members are likely to end up in one sort of asylum or another. In fact there is no evidence that homosexuals are generally physically different from heterosexuals. The basis of these ideas is, however, very interesting: it is the idea that because women like men, any man who is sexually attracted to another man must 'really' be a woman. Most theorists would hotly deny that any such crude reasoning had ever entered their heads, but, to the cynical reader, it is hard to escape the suspicion that it has more than passed through their minds.

The next set of theories was in terms of some genetic problem. There really is no reason to suppose this can be a cause: homosexuality does not run in families in the way that some genetic traits do.

Then there are theories of biochemical causes of homosexuality. The earliest ideas were in terms of homosexuals having reduced levels of testosterone (the male sex hormone) – again, the idea of homosexuals being less than real men. Other theorists have thought in terms of an excess of some female sex hormone. There is no hard evidence that the overwhelming majority of homosexuals differ at all biochemically from heterosexuals.

Then there are the ideas that homosexuals are suffering from psychiatric disturbances of various sorts. In fact there is evidence that homosexuals are more likely to be depressed and anxious than heterosexuals, but the more tolerant the environment they live in towards homosexuality, the smaller the difference is. Moreover, single people, including heterosexuals, are much more likely to be anxious or depressed than those with a partner. Far fewer homosexuals than heterosexuals are likely to be in a stable relationship with another person. Psychiatric disturbance in homosexuals seems to be a response to society's persecution and to being single, rather than a cause of homosexuality.

Early childhood relationships have also been the subject of close scrutiny, particularly from some psychoanalysts. The idea has been put forward that over-close relationships with mothers or very poor relationships with fathers produce homosexuals. It is the failure to resolve the Oedipus complex, that is, the child's inability to sort out his fears of his father and his unconscious sexual desires towards his mother, which is the root of homosexuality. Leaving aside the vexed issue of whether there is such a thing as the Oedipus complex, there is little evidence that families make homosexuals. This idea also is based on the concept that homosexuality is somehow a failure of adjustment, an immature way of behaving and feeling.

The truth of the matter may be that men and women probably have the in-built capacity to respond to a range of sexual stimuli. Everyone has the potential to be heterosexual or homosexual (which is different from saying that everyone *is* homosexual). Experiences during life, perhaps good homosexual experiences or bad heterosexual experiences, may mould a person's sexuality towards a homosexual orientation. People who have both good homosexual and good heterosexual experiences may find themselves with the capacity to respond to both men and women. Whatever the truth of the matter, it seems eminently clear that homosexuality is a normal variant of human sexuality, not a disease or a physical problem. If anyone doubts this they should consider just how frequent a sexual behaviour it is.

In 1948 Alfred Kinsey, Wardell Pomeroy and Clyde Martin published one of the most remarkable pieces of research of the century. The study was called *Sexual Behaviour in the Human Male*, more commonly referred to as the Kinsey Report, often by people who have not read it: the book runs to over 800 pages and is both dry reading and a mine of information about human sexuality.

What Kinsey and his colleagues did was to question 5,300 men in depth about their sex lives. What they found surprised them. Four per cent of their sample had been exclusively homosexual throughout their lives, ten per cent had been exclusively homosexual for at least three years between 16 and 55 and thirty-seven per cent overall of their sample had had at least one homosexual experience. A homosexual experience did not necessarily mean anal intercourse or oral sex but any experience where they reached orgasm.

The problem with Kinsey was that the sample used was not representative of the population at large. When Gagnon and Simon looked in 1973 at one group from the survey, college students, they found somewhat lower figures. Thirty per cent had had some homosexual experience at one time or another, mostly before the age of twenty, often an isolated experience, three per cent of the students had had a fair amount of both homosexual and heterosexual experiences and three per cent had always been totally homosexual. There is no way of telling, of course, whether college students are particularly typical of mankind in general either, but it is clear that a very large number of men have had at least some homosexual experience during their lives and six per cent of men have had considerable homosexual experience.

What the Kinsey data also showed was that there is little fixed in human sexuality. Many people's sexual orientation is fluid, it changes over the course of their lives, sometimes from homosexual to heterosexual, sometimes from heterosexual to homosexual. Quite a large number of men are attracted to both men and women. Kinsey himself suggested that sexuality was not something that could be divided as simply as saying that someone is homosexual, heterosexual or bisexual. Instead there is a continuum of sexuality from the man who has always been exclusively heterosexual to the man who has always been exclusively homosexual, with many gradations between.

It is a long time since Kinsey collected his data. No one knows whether there are now more homosexual men, or less, or whether things have stayed much the same. This is simply because there has never been another study like Kinsey's, much less a truly representative random study. The cost of mounting such a project and the difficulties in actually carrying it out are enormous. It is easy to guess at the problems involved if one imagines oneself quietly watching TV when a knock comes at the door and a man stands there ready to ask whether you are homosexual or heterosexual and how many orgasms you had last week. The tact required by the interviewer would verge on the superhuman.

THE LIVES OF HOMOSEXUAL MEN

The late 1960s were a time of sexual freedoms. Heterosexuals started to view their sexuality as an expression of their own individuality. More than that, there was money around and for the first time the young had that money. With the money came the opportunity to move from home, away from watchful parents and to the big cities, where anonymity allowed them to do what they wanted. The result was a revolution in sexual behaviour and attitudes. Morals were changing and for the first time there was the opportunity to take advantage of those changes.

It was not only heterosexuals who found life different:

homosexuals too felt the changes. Society was becoming rather more tolerant. They too were on the move. Gay men started to go to the big cities, to San Francisco and New York, to Amsterdam, to Copenhagen and to London. This concentration meant that it was easy to meet other gay men. Gay clubs mushroomed in all the big cities of America and Europe. Because gay men tend not to have families to drain their money, they began to become increasingly important economically to the cities they lived in. They had money in their pockets and they could spend it having fun. What has been called the 'pink economy' sprang up to provide that fun. With economic power came political power. Gay men began to assert their rights and 'gay pride' became the order of the day. Gay men began to get themselves elected to positions of political power, particularly in some big American cities, and no longer felt they had to hide their sexuality. It was not so everywhere, but in the Californian sun it was possible to imagine that a revolution in attitudes was just around the corner and everything was going to be all right.

The information we have about the sexual behaviour of gay men comes mostly from samples from the early 1970s of these young, geographically mobile, socially and politically active men. We have no idea how typical they are of gay men in general: it would take another Kinsey, asking different questions, to answer that. We do know that they were very different from other groups of gay men at the time, for instance those who meet their partners in public lavatories or older men. If they were different from these groups we know about, they were probably different from other, unknown groups in many aspects of their life-style, including the sexual aspects. It was among these men that AIDS first struck, and it is important to understand why.

It is a striking fact that these gay men had far more partners over a lifetime than heterosexuals. In a study of gay men in Baltimore and San Francisco in the 1970s, it turned out that ninety-four per cent of the gay men interviewed had had more than fifteen sexual partners compared with only twenty-one per cent of heterosexuals. Seventy-five per cent of homosexuals had had more than thirty sexual partners, but none of the heterosexuals studied. The more sexual partners you have the more likely you are to catch any sexually transmitted disease, and HTLV-III is no exception. Very few men had a monogamous sexual partnership with another man. Only ten per cent of homosexual men in a study by Bell and Weinberg were in a more or less monogamous relationship, and a further eighteen per cent had a partner but had many liaisons outside the relationship.

Why these particular gay men had more partners than heterosexuals is not entirely clear. It may be because gay men rarely marry and have children and so have less social ties to keep them with one partner, it may simply be a result of opportunity, but these cannot be the only explanations. Lesbian women, who are in a similar position as regards marriage and other social pressures, have far fewer sexual partners a year and are three times more likely to be in a stable, faithful relationship. Therefore the pattern is not just something about being homosexual, but something about being a homosexual man. It could be that these results tell us something about differences in attitudes to sex between men and women.

Studies by the present authors from a British sexually transmitted diseases clinic show a similar pattern of high numbers of sexual partners and low numbers of men in stable relationships: far more men express a wish to be in such relationships than are actually in them. Once again, though, such a sample is highly selective and no more typical of gay men in general than heterosexual clinic attenders are of heterosexuals in general.

There is no doubt also that all these studies greatly under-estimate the large numbers of men who are bisexual. Kinsey found that ten per cent of married men under 25 had at least some homosexual activity. There is a big overlap between the gay world and the heterosexual world, providing a clear path by which AIDS can move from homosexual men to heterosexuals (or vice versa).

HOMOSEXUALITY AND AIDS

The main reason that HTLV-III infection is particularly prevalent among gay men is simply that on average gay men tend to have more sexual partners than heterosexuals. For that same reason, gay men tend to have more sexually transmitted diseases of all sorts than heterosexuals. This is not to say that all gay men have more partners than all heterosexuals: many gay men have only a single sexual partner, many heterosexuals have many sexual partners.

There may also be other risk factors involved, in particular the specific sexual practices of gay men may put them at more risk. The most popular sexual activities of gay men are anal intercourse and oral sex. Anal intercourse may carry a particularly high risk of infection with HTLV-III. During anal intercourse there is almost always a certain amount of bleeding and this blood can carry the virus to the man inserting his penis while small tears can allow virus from semen to enter the body of the man receiving the penis. Contrary to myth, most gay men have both active and passive anal sex. The ano-rectal area has few defences against infection, unlike the vagina which has a tough elastic structure and a number of natural defence mechanisms against disease.

It looks as though another virus, hepatitis B which causes a liver infection, may be more easily passed on in anal sex than in vaginal sex and it may be that HTLV-III is also a little more easily passed on anally. But specific sexual practices are probably much less important than the sheer number of partners.

Another factor is simply that there are large numbers of gay men infected with the virus now: HTLV-III has a strong base in this group. For a heterosexual having intercourse with 40 other heterosexuals in a year the chance of one of those partners being infected are lower simply because fewer heterosexuals currently have the virus. In parts of America over sixty per cent of gay men are infected, in London perhaps twenty-five per cent of gay men may be. The risk of a gay man meeting an infected partner is therefore very high: on average in London every fourth man he meets will be infected.

Once a gay man has been infected with the virus his risk of actually going on to get AIDS is much higher than for any other group. Only about one per cent of infected haemophiliacs develop AIDS, whereas the figure for gay men is perhaps ten times higher. One element in this seems to be intercurrent sexually transmitted diseases, that is, catching new sexually transmitted diseases after already being infected with HTLV-III. Gay men have a much higher rate of other sexually transmitted diseases than those in other high-risk groups. These diseases seem to help the AIDS virus by challenging the immune system, in some infections by directly undermining it, and also perhaps sometimes by directly activating the virus.

HOW ARE GAY MEN RESPONDING TO AIDS?

AIDS was a great shock to many gay men. They had at last won the sexual freedoms that they had been denied for at least two thousand years and then suddenly they were all being taken away. It is hardly surprising that, early on, some gay men even imagined a government plot to get rid of them with a manufactured virus. In fact, no government on earth has the skill to build such a virus from scratch. Another suggestion was that the epidemic was an experiment in biological warfare gone wrong, a natural virus escaped from the lab. Anything less promising than HTLV-III as a biological warfare agent is difficult to imagine. It would only be of any use if the enemy troops could be guaranteed to have sex with each other, would take at least a year to work and anyway would only affect a minority.

The reaction of some sections of the press both in America and Europe did not help. Many reactionary people saw AIDS as a 'gay plague', as something that gay men had brought on themselves. It was even argued by some of the more extreme anti-homosexual lobby that it was some sort of punishment from God. This bizarre concept seems never to have been taken to its logical conclusion by its supporters. Presumably they would have to argue that toxaemia of pregnancy is a punishment for heterosexuality, or that small-pox is a punishment for being alive. It also does not seem to have dawned on them that if God had sent down a punishment, he would presumably not have sent researchers to find a cure.

Gay men themselves were caught in something of a trap. Having just grown accustomed to the freedoms they had fought so long for they were loath to see them snatched away, and the changes in life-style needed to reduce the risk of infection were enormous. Consequently gay men did not always act as rapidly as they might have done. In Europe there was more warning than in America, where AIDS was well established before it was even known that it was caused by an infection. There was little anyone could have done in that situation. Gay men in Europe, however, were able to watch the disease spread through America. They were able to follow its progress in the gay press, in the newspapers and on television. Few people acted early enough to try to limit their own risk of infection. Undoubtedly many gay men hoped that the virus would not spread to Europe and that the problem would simply go away. It is hard to be unsympathetic to this very human response.

In both America and Europe some people reacted rapidly. The London-based AIDS charity the Terrence Higgins Trust was formed as early as 1982 and made strong efforts to educate gay men in changing their life-style to reduce the risk of infection. For a long time they were simply a voice in the wilderness. Some people prudently listened and followed their advice, most did not. It was only when people found their friends dying of AIDS that the warnings began to take effect. There is nothing peculiar to being gay about these reactions. If AIDS starts to spread widely among heterosexuals there is little doubt that exactly the same thing will happen. Heterosexuals also will respond too slowly.

Today many gay men have changed their sexual behaviour to reduce their risk of infection or, if infected, to prevent others from getting the virus from them. The changes have often been quite striking. Mostly they have drastically reduced the number of partners they have. Unfortunately this is not having the desired effect of limiting spread. The reason is simple. It is like running downhill with a snowball rolling after you: you have to go faster and faster just to say the same distance ahead. As men have cut their number of partners the risk of any given partner's being infected has risen.

This can be seen if we take an arithmetically simple example, not reflecting the true figures but easy to follow. If ten per cent of men are infected with a sexually transmitted virus and a man has twenty partners a year he will, on average, have two infected partners a year. If the percentage of infected men rises to forty per cent and he cuts his number of sexual partners to five a year, he will still, on average, have two infected partners a year. This is exactly what has been happening with HTLV-III in both America and Europe.

Gay men have cut their number of sexual partners to something around about a quarter over the last four years. In the same period the number of infected gay men has risen four fold. The net result is that they have not reduced their risk of infection, even though they have made huge changes in their lives.

It is not a change in numbers of sexual partners that will make a difference, it is a change to safer sexual practices. Unfortunately many gay men find such sexual practices less fun than what they have been used to. It is easy to imagine the response of the average heterosexual couple to being told that they can no longer have vaginal intercourse or oral sex but should stick to mutual masturbation and body rubbing. Even the use of condoms can be a problem. The issues of preventing sexual transmission are covered in more detail in Chapter 6.

For once it is not society that is persecuting gay men, it is sheer bad luck. With no cure or treatment available at the moment the only thing that gay men can do is to look after their own health. Doing so is not an easy option but it is one they must take if they are to avoid the serious consequences of infection with HTLV-III.

Chapter Eight

THE RISK GROUPS II: Haemophiliacs, Heroin Users and Heterosexuals

Gay men are the main risk group for AIDS at the moment, but there are others. This chapter looks at·some of those others and the problems they face.

HAEMOPHILIACS

When most of us injure ourselves and bleed the bleeding soon stops because our blood clots and forms a seal to prevent further bleeding. The process of clotting is a very complicated one involving many different elements, or factors. Haemophiliacs lack one of these factors, Factor VIII. A few people lack another factor, Factor IX, but Factor VIII deficiency is far more common. Because haemophiliacs lack these factors their blood does not clot properly: if they start to bleed they bleed for much longer. It is not external bleeding which is the main problem. If they knock themselves they may bleed into their joints, causing great pain and often deformity.

The severity of haemophilia varies. Most haemophiliacs have some Factor VIII in their blood. Those who have more than about 5% of the normal levels are usually only mildly affected and suffer problems only with fairly major injury.

The worst cases have less than 2% of the normal levels of Factor VIII and, without treatment, suffer major problems.

Classical haemophilia is the result of a defective gene. The gene is passed on by women to their children but only the males develop the condition, except in the rare circumstances where a haemophiliac man and a female carrier have children. Haemophiliac men are unable to pass on the condition to their children, but their sisters may do so. Haemophiliac men can pass on the defective gene to their daughters, who are protected against its effects, but not to their sons.

The lives of severe haemophiliacs were at one time lives of pain and suffering. Life expectancy was short, permanent disability inevitable. It must have seemed like a dream come true when a treatment was found, not a cure, but a way to reduce the symptoms. The answer was simply to take blood from healthy donors and to extract the missing Factor VIII from this blood. If the haemophiliac injured himself he could inject himself with some of this Factor VIII and the bleeding would stop.

The Factor VIII concentrates that most haemophiliacs use are prepared on an enormous scale. Five thousand pints of blood are pooled and large amounts of concentrate prepared in one batch. These batches are then broken down into small amounts and sent out to haemophiliacs. With the introduction of concentrates two things rapidly became obvious: firstly, that it was little short of a miracle for haemophiliacs who could at last lead a normal life; secondly, that it was a blessing not without its darker side. The problem was that if thousands of pints of blood were pooled together, some of them were likely to be infected with a variety of viruses. When haemophiliacs used Factor VIII they tended to catch these viruses.

The first virus to cause concern was hepatitis B, a rather dangerous virus which causes liver damage and can kill.

Testing blood used in preparing Factor VIII to make as sure as possible that it was clear of hepatitis B provided a partial solution, but occasionally infected blood failed to show up and many haemophiliacs have been infected with hepatitis B virus. Even so, when you can look forward to a life of disability and early death without Factor VIII the risk of hepatitis seems an acceptable one.

When HTLV-III appeared in the early 1980s this too began to get into the Factor VIII supply. No one knew early on that AIDS was an infectious disease, and even when they found out, it was initially impossible to test for HTLV-III. The result was that many haemophiliacs have been infected with this virus. America was and still is the world's largest producer of commercial Factor VIII, much of which was exported, some of it to the UK and Europe. America is of course also the place where the earliest cases of AIDS appeared in the West. Many British haemophiliacs used American Factor VIII and became infected. However, many haemophiliacs who have used only UK concentrates have also been infected.

Britain is moving towards self-sufficiency in Factor VIII production, largely as a result of worries about HTLV-III. All the blood going into British Factor VIII is screened to make sure it is as far as possible free of the virus. The Factor VIII is then heat treated, essentially cooked for many hours to kill the virus. Similar steps are being taken in America for US Factor VIII concentrate. We can hope that in future there will be no more cases of HTLV-III infection in haemophiliacs. Unfortunately that still leaves many haemophiliacs who are already infected with the virus.

BLOOD TRANSFUSION RECIPIENTS

In both America and Europe small numbers of people have been infected after they have been given blood for operations or accidents that has been infected with the virus. The number of people infected has been tiny compared to the number of people having transfusions, but in every country in the Western world the blood transfusion services have taken strong action to make sure that the blood supply is safe.

The earliest step they took was to ask people who thought that they might be infected with the virus, or anyone in a high-risk group, not to give blood. Even people who are in high-risk groups who have been tested and found to be negative should not give blood. There is a small chance of the test results being wrong, and they could, of course, become infected after the time of the test. When tests for HTLV-III antibodies became available the blood transfusion services of the West introduced routine screening of all blood. Currently every pint of blood passing through the National Blood Transfusion Service in Britain is tested to make sure that it is not infected with the virus. Similar arrangements exist in most of Europe and in America.

The combination of these two measures should mean that no one should risk being infected with this virus in the future through blood donations.

Unfortunately blood is a very emotive subject and people do not necessarily understand the issues involved. In America, in particular, many people are demanding the right to use their own blood if they need a transfusion. Suppose they want to have a routine operation in the future. They arrange to give regular donations of their own blood which is specially labelled and stored, then when they have the operation they can be transfused with their own blood. Others insist on having donations only from their relatives. Most European blood transfusion services have strongly resisted this practice.

It is extremely expensive and complex to administer such a system and if everyone insisted on it most blood transfusion services would collapse. Much of the need for blood transfusions comes from emergency procedures, accidents, operations carried out at short notice and so on, where prior storage is just not possible. It is also quite unnecessary given the precautions outlined above. Taking blood from your relatives is even more of a problem. You may think you know about their sexual and personal lives, but can you be entirely sure? A relative asked to give blood may be put in the awkward position of either donating or having to admit to being bisexual or gay.

Since the introduction of testing of blood donations for HTLV-III the number of people giving blood in the UK has fallen sharply in some areas. A few of the people who have stopped giving blood were in high-risk groups, but it seems that some people have become afraid that they can catch AIDS by donating (as opposed to being given) blood. This is not true. The use of sterile procedures and disposable equipment for taking blood donations means that it is not possible to catch HTLV-III by this means. Donors can be reassured that they need have nothing to fear. It is important that everyone not in a high-risk group should give blood if possible, to make up for the shortfall.

INTRAVENOUS DRUG USERS

Intravenous drug users are those who inject themselves, usually with heroin. They are at very high risk of getting AIDS.

If the seed pods of the oriental poppy, *Papaver somniferum*, are cut when they are ripe a milky juice seeps out. This milky juice dries and solidifies into a dark mass of crude opium. For centuries men have used opium to kill pain and to bring a sense of well-being. Opium itself is a complex mass of chemicals called, collectively, the opiates. The most widely used opiate today is heroin, prepared chemically from opium. The drug is a powerful pain-killer, but is little used in medicine: its main market is as an illegal drug.

The cells of the brain do not actually touch one another, there are tiny gaps between them across which the cells signal to one another by sending out minute amounts of chemicals. These chemicals are called, not surprisingly, transmitters: they transmit information from brain cell to brain cell. There may be a hundred different brain transmitters, there may be thousands, no one really knows. But one group of transmitters, the endorphins, are especially interesting because chemically they are very similar to the opiate drugs. It seems that heroin probably gets its effects by mimicking the endorphin brain transmitters. The endorphins control pain. Therefore heroin, by imitating their effects in the brain, can also control pain. But the endorphins not only reduce physical pain, they also seem to reduce emotional pain, anxiety, fear and all the punishing things of the world. As with the endorphins, so with heroin: taking it reduces people's bad feelings about themselves and the world and by doing so increases the pleasure they feel. It is hardly surprising that many who are unhappy or miserable should turn to drugs such as heroin for an escape from the world.

The problem is that heroin is very addictive. Although it is not a particularly dangerous drug when taken in small amounts, it is easy to overdose on it and it does have its side-effects: it causes constipation, suppresses coughing – an important bodily defence – and reduces sexual drive. In larger doses it can suppress respiration and kill. But the main medical problem with heroin is a psychological one. It stops people caring so much about what they are doing and, in some cases, saps their drive to do anything except take the drug.

105

However it is the fact that the drug is illegal which is the major problem for many heroin users. Because they rapidly become addicted they need the drug every day. They also develop tolerance, that is, they need gradually to take more of the drug for it to take effect. Because heroin is so expensive only a few people can support their habit by legal means. Others are forced to turn to selling the drug themselves, to crime or to prostitution in order to finance their habit. There is also the ever-present fear of being caught.

In parts of the United States, in New York for instance, it is illegal not only to take heroin but even to possess a syringe with which to inject it. Heroin users therefore go to 'shooting galleries', hideaways like the old opium dens, where they can borrow or hire a syringe. Hygiene is non-existent and the same syringe has been employed by many different users. These users not only inject themselves with the drug but they may engage in 'pumping', moving their blood in and out of their veins. The result is a syringe heavily contaminated with blood. Often that blood contains viruses such as hepatitis B: these days it is often infected with HTLV-III.

Needle-sharing is not limited to New York. Even in Britain, where it is not illegal to have a syringe, many users share syringes with other people. In some work by John Green with Geraldine Mulleady, it was found that over half of a group of British drug users shared syringes with other people from time to time, either because they had forgotten their own, because they were sharing a fix of the drug, or simply to be sociable. Most heroin users will share at some stage in their lives, particularly early on, before they have their own syringes. Therefore it is young, new drug-users who are most at risk. As drug addiction rates rise they constitute the largest group of users.

It is needle-sharing, not heroin, that gives drug users AIDS. There is no need to persuade them to give up heroin in order to reduce their risk of contracting HTLV-III, it is only necessary to persuade them to keep to their own syringe and not share it with others. Unfortunately there are a number of difficulties in achieving this aim. Drug users are not a group of people noted for looking after their general health, so persuading them to be sensible is not always easy, and there are other problems.

Drug addiction is almost as much of a problem as AIDS in many Western countries. The main approach to treatment of drug users in Europe and America is methadone reduction. The patient is put on to a synthetic opiate, methadone, then the dose they are given is gradually reduced. This allows them to stop taking opiates without the withdrawal effects of suddenly stopping. (These withdrawal effects can be quite uncomfortable although not quite so dramatic as they are portrayed in films and books.) Methadone is a drug taken by mouth. There is therefore a conflict between drug clinics offering an oral drug and encouraging their patients to use clean syringes and avoid needle-sharing. Results of methadone reduction programmes are not generally particularly good, and the majority of patients on them drift back on to heroin. On the other hand, they do help some people and it is difficult to find alternatives that can be carried out on a large scale.

If drug users are to stick to using their own syringes they need to be able to get a clean syringe when they need one. In some parts of the world getting a syringe is not just difficult, it is illegal. Elsewhere, in Britain for instance, the dispensing of syringes is a matter of discretion for the pharmacist, but it is still fairly difficult to find a pharmacist who will actually sell them. Most governments and professionals in the field are not keen to make syringes more freely available because they feel it will encourage people to take drugs. This seems a rather short-sighted attitude, since most people who want them already manage to get syringes one way or another, usually by sharing them and catching HTLV-III and hepatitis B in the process. The system in the Netherlands seems the best in this respect. Addicts are encouraged to bring in an old syringe and to swap it for a clean one. At the same time they are encouraged not to share and given health education. If a similar system were adopted elsewhere it might just stop the spread of the problem.

AIDS in drug users is not a problem limited to that particular group. Some drug-using men and many drug-using women turn to prostitution as a source of income to buy drugs. In doing so they provide an ideal way for the virus to spread into other groups in the population.

PAEDIATRIC AIDS

AIDS among children is an emotive subject. There have been many cases across the world. The child receives the virus from a mother who is infected, either in the womb or during the birth. HTLV-III is also secreted in breast milk. It seems possible that an uninfected child may subsequently be infected by suckling at its mother's breast if she is infected. Not every infected mother will give birth to an infected child, perhaps only 50% will do so, but infected babies are particularly at risk of going on to develop AIDS. There seem to be two reasons. Firstly, their immune systems are immature and they easily fall prey to the virus. Secondly, the young baby is meeting for the first time a whole world of infections and chemicals which keep the immune system they do have in a constant state of activity. These are just the conditions in which the virus can flourish. Although the rate of AIDS in infected babies is difficult to be sure about, it may be as high as 50%, certainly much higher than in adults.

It is not only the baby who is at risk if the mother is seropositive, the mother also is at risk because the changes in the immune system which accompany pregnancy allow the virus an ideal opportunity to get a good hold. The only sensible course of action for a seropositive pregnant woman is to have the pregnancy terminated for her own sake; this is not advice that most women are happy to hear.

Women who are infected should not have children, at least until we find a way of controlling the virus. Even women whose partners are infected should not become pregnant by their partners: the ejaculation which makes them pregnant may also be the one that infects them. There are of course ways in which women can conceive in these circumstances: artificial insemination by donor is one way (semen donors are always screened for the virus). Few women find this the ideal way of having a child – they want the baby of their partner, not of someone else – but there is nothing anyone can do to help at the moment.

If HTLV-III spreads widely in the heterosexual population, paediatric AIDS will become a major problem. It raises the issue of whether all pregnant women should be screened for the virus, as they are for syphilis for instance. AIDS is, however, rather different. It is so emotive a subject that many pregnant women will be very upset by the prospect of being tested, but they must be told they are being tested for the reasons outlined in Chapter 11. The answer at the moment seems to be to test only those women who are in high-risk groups, or whose partners are in high-risk groups. The woman may not, of course, know that her partner is bisexual, so it may be that the only course of action is to interview all fathers early in the pregnancy and get the information directly from them.

HETEROSEXUALS

The thing the press fears, and which governments fear above all else, is the spread of HTLV-III among heterosexuals. If such a spread takes place the potential numbers of people who could be infected will rise by a factor of at least ten. But are they really at risk?

AIDS is no respecter of sexual preferences. In Africa it is a heterosexual disease, but there are special factors in Africa. In America and Europe there have been many cases of heterosexual AIDS where women in particular have caught the virus from partners in high-risk groups, bisexual men, haemophiliacs and those who have caught the virus through blood donations. They did not always know that their partner was in a high-risk group. It is also possible that some men have caught the virus from heterosexual contact, particularly with drug-using prostitutes. However the percentage of AIDS cases accounted for by heterosexual contact has not changed much in America over the past three years.

Some researchers have taken the view that the virus is less easily spread in vaginal intercourse than in anal intercourse, citing studies which show that, while a male sexual partner of another man has roughly a 50% chance of becoming infected, only 10% of female sexual partners of infected men seem to become infected. This evidence needs to be treated with extreme caution; most of it is drawn from small studies using the female partners of haemophiliacs, and it may well be inapplicable to other groups. Information from artificial insemination by donor and from female sexual partners of bisexual men suggests that women are at higher risk, perhaps just as great as in male-to-male transmission.

Whatever the relative risks of anal and vaginal sex, there is no doubt that women can be infected by contact with men and men can be infected by contact with women. There is no real reason why AIDS should not spread amongst heterosexuals. At the moment the virus has a low base in heterosexuals in the West, that is, few heterosexuals are infected and so the spread among heterosexuals is likely to be slow. If that base starts to rise, if more people start to become infected, the picture could change very quickly indeed. Once the spread started to accelerate it would be very difficult to stop the process.

The way in which women become infected has been the subject of much debate. Some people have alleged that heterosexual anal intercourse is the main risk factor. It is quite clear from Africa that vaginal intercourse is the main route of transmission in heterosexual sex. It has also been suggested that the vagina needs to be damaged for transmission to occur, perhaps by small lesions which the woman would not even notice. On the other hand, there are many cells in the vagina and cervix which lie close to the surface and which are of a type that could be infected with HTLV-III, including T-cells and close relatives of T-cells. There is every reason to suppose that vaginal intercourse without any damage, and at any time of the menstrual cycle, could lead to infection of the woman. The exact mechanism by which men are infected in vaginal intercourse remains uncertain but the virus is present in cervical and vaginal secretions.

The people most at risk are those with multiple sexual partners. Many men are, or have been, bisexual, so that women with many sexual partners stand a good chance of meeting one. Of course a single partner could infect a woman, but the fewer partners she has the lower the risk of meeting someone who is infected. The answer to the problem is actually fairly straightforward. Men and women starting a relationship with someone, or having a casual affair with someone they know nothing about, should always use a condom, preferably with some back-up method of contraception, the pill or the cap for instance, in case the sheath breaks. Condoms are far less of a problem in vaginal intercourse than in anal intercourse, where conventional condoms may break rather more often. They are actually designed for vaginal intercourse, where the mechanical strains involved are much less than in anal sex.

A return to the use of condoms would not protect against HTLV-III only but also against the wart virus, papilloma, which seems to be the main cause of the upsurge of cervical cancer among younger women. It would also offer some protection against herpes, gonorrhoea, syphilis, non-specific urethritis and a wide range of sexually transmitted diseases. A packet of condoms should be in the handbag of every sexually active young woman and the jacket pocket of every sexually active young man. They may not be aesthetic but they really do ensure safer sex.

PROSTITUTES

One special risk category of heterosexuals is prostitutes. As mentioned in Chapter 3, Central African prostitutes have very high rates of HTLV-III infections. In the United States many prostitutes are infected with the virus, usually because they are also intravenous drug users. There is no evidence that UK prostitutes are currently infected with the virus on a large scale, except those who are also intravenous drug users: the size of this group is hard to estimate, and there have been cases of non-drug-using UK prostitutes being infected. In theory prostitutes could form a reservoir for the transmission of the virus into the heterosexual community. This does not seem to have happened yet in Europe, but in Africa it seems to have been one of the main contributory causes of the spread of AIDS. What will happen in the West depends on a number of factors which are difficult to assess.

Many New York prostitutes are infected with HTLV-III because they are also drug addicts, but there is no evidence that they are spreading the virus on a large scale. There seem to be two reasons why not. Firstly oral sex and manual manipulation seem to be the main sexual activities at the lower end of the US prostitution market, in which most drug-using prostitutes operate. Secondly, there is a very high rate of usage of condoms by prostitutes in this group.

In Britain the situation is somewhat similar. At the lower end of the market prostitutes will try if possible to bring the man to orgasm manually. If this is not agreeable they will insist as far as possible on the use of a condom. Oral sex seems to be much less common as a customer request in Britain and less prostitutes seem prepared to perform it. At the upper end of the market, among 'escort girls' who work hotels for instance, the situation is rather different. Prices are higher and the prostitute will sometimes not be able to insist on the use of a condom. For an extra fee the prostitute will often agree to 'extras', especially anal intercourse which is much in demand from Middle Eastern and Mediterranean clients. The situation in Britain is quite similar to that in Europe in general, although there are variations from country to country, especially in those countries where the state tries to regulate prostitution. Unfortunately it is impossible to say whether the experience from America is at all applicable to Western Europe.

Chapter Nine

PEOPLE WHO ARE INFECTED BY HTLV-III

For people who are HTLV-III infected the first contact with the hospital or clinic is usually a surprising one. They may have decided to come along to be tested because they have been feeling unwell, or because they know they have been in contact with someone they fear may have been infected or simply because they suspect that they are in a high-risk group and feel that they would like to know.

The first surprise is that before they are tested the clinic will try to make sure that they have really thought through whether they want the test.

From the clinic's point of view the test is something of a Pandora's box. If it turns out that a patient is infected with the virus there is currently nothing, medically, the clinic can do about it. There is no treatment. The test does not tell them whether the patient has got AIDS or not (that is decided on the basis of the patient's symptoms and other tests). It does not tell them whether the patient will go on to get AIDS or will stay well in the future. In fact it quite often tells them little that is very helpful.

The clinic will be well aware that regardless of the test result they are likely to offer the same advice about safer sex and about issues like not donating blood. For people in high-risk groups the same advice will protect them from getting the virus and prevent them from passing it on to others. Regardless of test results, the person in a high-risk group should never give blood anyway. There is always a small chance of a test result being wrong. If the person has been recently infected the antibodies that the test looks for will not yet have been produced, or the person may be negative on the test and then go out and get infected the following day. Therefore neither a positive nor a negative result will help the clinic very much in advising people. They want to try to inform patients of the risks and get them to consider making certain changes in their lives, and the test results are almost irrelevant to that task.

The clinic is also aware of the tremendous problems which being tested and found to be infected can bring. For example, it is currently almost impossible to get life insurance, an endowment mortgage, or anything else that depends on health for a person known to be infected. Applicants for insurance must disclose all the material facts to the insurance company: if any are concealed and the insurance company finds out, they will refuse to pay up in the event of illness. Being infected also presents difficulties in filling in health questionnaires for new employment. This can mean not being able to change jobs.

More than that, the test results can lead to a great deal of extra worry. Most people coming to be tested would be only too happy to hear that they were not infected, but few people really want to find out that they are infected. When told, they usually become very anxious, often distraught. They may become depressed or panic. All these things can be handled but it takes patient counselling, often over a few weeks, before those who are infected come to terms with it.

It is a tribute to people's ability to face up to difficulties that virtually everyone does come to terms with a positive test result if they are dealt with well by the clinic, if they are offered appropriate counselling and if they are given all the information they need to understand what is happening to them. Self-help groups often add greatly to the process of adjustment, because it is helpful for people to meet others in their own situation, to see how they have coped and to see that they are in good health.

Ultimately it is the decision of patients, not of the clinic, whether they should be tested. That is as it should be. Many people in high-risk groups do want to be tested because they dislike the uncertainty of not knowing. If that is what they want they will be tested, but it must be an informed decision. That is why many clinics lay great stress on 'pre-counselling' people coming for the test, that is, getting them to think through the issues involved.

There are some situations where it is definitely helpful to be tested. It might be helpful for a doctor trying to make a diagnosis, although this is much rarer than might at first appear. Knowing that someone is infected with HTLV-III does not necessarily mean that any symptoms that happen to be present are caused by the virus. It is helpful in the case of a woman who fears that she may have been exposed to the virus and wants to become pregnant. Perhaps a haemophiliac wants to know what sexual precautions he needs to take. Since he is not likely to pick up the virus sexually, his situation is rather different from that of, say, a gay man. Even in these cases there is some degree of difficulty. Four per cent of people with negative test results seem to be infected with the virus, so there is some risk which needs to be discussed with the patient.

A few people argue that members of high-risk groups should be positively encouraged to be tested. They argue that by doing so we can try to halt the spread of the disease. This argument really doesn't hold water when it is closely ex-amined. For a start, whatever encouragement is offered the experience in both Europe and America is that only a minority of people in high-risk groups will come forward to be tested, certainly not enough to make much real impact on the spread of the disease. Secondly, of course, it is not the test which prevents the spread of HTLV-III, it is changes in life-style, and people can be offered exactly the same advice whether they are tested or not. Another argument sometimes put forward for testing is that it helps to protect health staff. The argument has little merit. This issue is discussed in detail in Chapter 11.

It is, in fact, a good idea for people who know they are infected, or simply fear they might be, to tell their doctor and dentist. This should allow the professional to keep a close eye on their health and to be in a better position to advise them if they become unwell. Unfortunately some doctors and dentists react with blind panic. For people who fear that they are infected but cannot be sure of the reaction of their doctor or dentist the answer is simple: change them. Any doctor or dentist who is going to react badly in those circumstances is not worth staying with in any case. Local sexually transmitted disease clinics or local voluntary groups can usually help in offering advice.

When someone does decide to be tested, the wait for the result is a very anxious time for most patients. Although in theory the test can be done and analysed in a single day, few laboratories have the facilities to be able to respond so quickly. So patients are given a time to come back. Some people get a very nice surprise when they find they are negative on the test, that they probably have not been infected. They are still given the same advice on how to stay negative, of course.

For the person who is positive, who is infected, the outcome is very different. The majority, however much they may have expected it, are profoundly shocked. They can hardly believe the result. They tend immediately to think that they have AIDS, however carefully it has been explained to them what the test means before they are tested. It is at this point that careful counselling is usually necessary from someone who is in command of all the facts.

For someone who is positive (and for all who feel that they are at risk, even those who are negative) quite large changes in life-style have to be made. Sexual habits have to be changed. No one at the clinic either can or will want to force changes on anyone. However, once all the facts have been explained to them most people do not want to risk passing on the virus to anyone else. They have to be helped to think through the enormous implications of this virus for them personally.

Just to take one example, sex is not just a matter of orgasms; it provides far more for people whether heterosexual or homosexual. It provides closeness, a way of getting to know people very well, it provides comfort and physical contact and it sometimes presents a route whereby people eventually settle down and form a stable relationship. A positive test need not hinder any of these things. Enjoyable sexual activity is still possible but it needs imagination and foresight.

Some people find it presents particular problems. The young haemophiliac boy who has never had a sexual relationship, for example: how is he to deal with his first relationships with women knowing that he has to restrict his sexual activities and must tell any potential sexual partner what has happened? The gay man who has to discuss with potential partners at an early stage the fact that he will only have safe sex: how will he achieve this, at a party or in a bar, without frightening them off?

But the greatest problem that someone who is infected faces is not medical. It is ignorance and fear. Although such a person presents no risk to others, except sexually or through blood, few people will understand this. The newspapers, radio and television tell a very different story. Directly or by implication they tell the story of a dreadfully infectious virus which is a risk to anyone and everyone, of infected people being akin to the lepers of the Middle Ages, to be shunned and feared. No one working in the field recognises the description that the media all too often give. They know that the virus simply is not like that. It is, however, very difficult to get that message across sometimes. One journalist on a national newspaper told us that his editor simply would not print anything about AIDS that was good news, short of a cure. For that reason most people infected with the virus are currently well advised not to tell a lot of other people that they are infected. There are some people they may want or need to tell, but they would be unwise to tell all their workmates, for instance, unless they can be very, very certain of their reaction.

One of our cases illustrates the problem very well. A man had a positive blood test for HTLV-III. He told a colleague, who turned out to be rather less than discreet. When he returned to work he found that his desk had been moved out of the office he shared and placed in a small cubby-hole in a corridor and his workmates had bought him his own kettle so that he could have coffee separately from them. He also noticed that people no longer came to see him, but rang him if possible; if they did have to see him, they tended to stand at least twenty feet away and shout. Understandably all this started to depress him after a while. He was able to sort matters out by explaining the true facts to two of his more sympathetic workmates who managed to persuade the others that they were not at risk. If he had been a little less articulate and persuasive he might even now be sitting with his lonely cup of coffee in the corridor, a victim of quite unfounded prejudices.

Many people who have the test and turn out to be infected feel quite out of control and helpless. They feel there is nothing they can do to help themselves. In fact there are many things they can do. Firstly, they can avoid getting any new sexually transmitted diseases. These are probable co-factors in the development of AIDS, in other words they tend to make someone's prospects much worse. Secondly, they can avoid 'live' vaccines if they have a vaccination. Chapter 12 explains the different types of vaccine available. The live type may cause problems in someone who is HTLV-III infected and should be avoided. Of course the average person is not going to know whether a vaccine that they are about to be given is live or killed, but the person giving the vaccine will know and they should be told that only killed vaccine should be used.

It also makes sense for people who are infected to look after their general health. It makes sense to eat a well-balanced diet. There is no need to go on any special 'HTLV-III diet', indeed, there is no such thing, nor are there any foodstuffs which a person with HTLV-III, or AIDS for that matter, should avoid. Most people, regardless of whether they are infected or not, would benefit from a varied diet with plenty of fresh foods, which is not to say that someone who is infected cannot have convenience foods, but they should not constitute the bulk of anyone's diet.

Getting plenty of rest and relaxation is also advisable. Most people lead very stressful lives these days. A little stress is no bad thing, and it is unavoidable, but most people have areas of their lives in which they can reduce the stress they experience. Often they can rearrange their work so that they are less pressured, and there may be areas in their private lives where they can do the same thing. Most people would benefit from an hour a day just sitting reading or listening to music.

Regular exercise is also a good thing. This does not mean that those people infected with the virus who have taken no exercise for twenty years should suddenly go out and play five hard games of squash a week. The squash is more likely to kill them than the virus. However some activity that the person enjoys, maybe a sport, but perhaps just going for a walk every day or going swimming, could provide exercise.

It is also important for someone who is infected to maintain a positive attitude to life. Most people postpone their pleasures because they are too busy doing what they feel they must do to do what they want to do. It is helpful for someone who is infected actually to plan to make life more pleasurable.

All these positive health steps are good advice for anyone and certainly would do no one any harm. There are good grounds for thinking that some, or maybe all of them, could help a person with HTLV-III infection, even though there is no hard scientific evidence at the moment that they do. At the very least they make life more fun. It is important to recognise that the same advice that can be offered to those who are infected applies to those who feel that they are in a high-risk group, even though they have not been tested.

It is also important to recognise that many of those who come forward for testing are not in any high-risk group and are simply worried; indeed, they are called the 'worried well' by clinics. Each era has a disease that people fear above all others. In Victorian times anyone who had symptoms they did not understand immediately feared that they might have tuberculosis, then an incurable condition. Until recently cancer has been the major fear. Today, because of the publicity surrounding it, AIDS is the great fear. The symptoms of anxiety are so striking and dramatic that many people are simply unable to comprehend that dizziness, shortness of breath, pounding heart, aches and pains and even faintness can be attributable to something so simple. The more they worry about AIDS, the more ill they feel. If they become depressed as a result of their worries they may suffer from lethargy and malaise. Sometimes the symptoms produced by anxiety look surprisingly like some of those seen in HTLV-III infection, so much so that we have called the condition 'pseudo-AIDS' in our publications. A review of the patient's history and a simple examination will show that it is anxiety, not HTLV-III, which is the problem. Naturally the outlook and treatment are very different: no one ever died of this sort of anxiety.

It is hardly surprising that the worried well tend to turn up for testing. Often all that is required is a conversation with someone who can explain the situation to them and offer practical advice on overcoming their anxieties. Like anyone else, they are entitled to the test if they want it and are often amazed to find that the result is negative, even though the clinic staff knew it would be.

Chapter Ten

PEOPLE WITH AIDS

Most people have only the haziest idea what an AIDS patient looks like, vaguely imagining a gaunt, skeletal, sick-looking person confined to a hospital bed, waiting to die. Nothing could be further from the truth. You may well have sat next to an AIDS patient on the train or know one quite well without being aware of the illness. The majority of people with AIDS live reasonably normal lives in the community, as indeed they should. They are no risk to anyone else and for most of the time they are well.

The AIDS sufferer who only has Kaposi's sarcoma on the skin of his arms or legs suffers very little physical inconvenience: it is not usually painful. If it is on the face it is sometimes unsightly, but the use of a masking make-up can often help. Therefore most patients who only have KS are looked after as out-patients and are likely to be admitted to hospital only if the KS spreads, for instance to the internal organs, if they are being brought in for some form of treatment, or if they develop other problems of some sort.

AIDS patients who get opportunistic infections usually have a rather different pattern of admissions. They are likely to have a number of spells in hospital when they are actually ill. For instance, many people with AIDS develop pneumocystis carinii pneumonia (PCP), a chest infection, and while they have the infection they often feel very unwell.

They are admitted into hospital, the PCP is treated and they are then discharged. They may come in again if the problem recurs or if a new one arises. Again they are treated and discharged. The result is that they spend most of their time getting on with their lives with a few intermittent spells in hospital. During one of the admissions, if the infection they are suffering from cannot be brought under control, they may die, but there is not usually a long period of terminal illness as such. Dying itself is usually much less feared by people with AIDS than the possibility of dying in pain or of dying alone: in this they are similar to many people who are facing possible death. With good hospital care they should not have to fear pain, which can be controlled. Nor should they need to fear dying alone. A good hospital should make it possible for relatives or a lover to be with them and the hospital staff should always be on hand.

Although AIDS is often thought of as an invariably fatal disease there are people alive and in reasonable health who have had it for three or more years. Further than that we cannot say; the disease has not been around long enough. For any patient it is never possible to give a life expectancy, to say, 'You have six months to live' or 'You have two years to live.' It would not be a good idea if we could, and we cannot. We have seen people come into hospital with opportunistic infections who were not expected to survive the night, then seen them being discharged two or three weeks later, quite recovered.

The issue for many AIDS patients is not so much the problem of dying as the problem of living. A large part of that is the way that society reacts to them. The average man in the street sees an AIDS patient as a dreadful potential source of infection: the disease brings out people's deepest irrational fears of contamination and sickness. In fact, there is no risk of catching HTLV-III from an AIDS patient through everyday contact: the virus is not airborne, is not passed on by touching and cannot be caught from cups, plates or door handles. The only ways it can be caught are through either sexual contact or blood. Despite the careful and detailed advice from medical advisers it is hard even for the average AIDS patient to keep this in mind. Some newspapers carry stories which make AIDS appear to be like the Black Death. As a result many AIDS sufferers quite unreasonably feel a risk to others and shut themselves away.

There are often other worries for the person with AIDS. As well as the fear that a partner may also be infected, there is the worry of whether the partner will be able to cope with the patient's death, will have enough money to live on and about the loved one's future. It is vital for anyone with AIDS to make a will and there are particular problems for gay AIDS sufferers. The law does not recognise the rights of gay partners and only a will can ensure their rights.

How well someone with AIDS copes with the diagnosis depends vitally on the response of those around, not only partner and friends but also the hospitals and clinics concerned.

Chapter Eleven

HTLV-III AND HEALTH CARE

The appearance of HTLV-III infection has presented a number of problems, both clinical and financial, for health care in Europe and America, and is likely to do so even more in the future. In Africa the problems are even greater: the burden on the health care systems of developing countries is enormous.

It is clear that the virus itself provides little risk to health care staff. The virus was not identified until 1983 and in the early days of the epidemic AIDS was not even known to be caused by an infectious agent, with the result that health care staff took no special precautions whatsoever in dealing with patients. They operated on them, dealt with their body fluids and cared for them in exactly the same way that they would for any other patient with a non-infectious condition. No one developed AIDS or HTLV-III infection as a result of their normal work.

Today in the United States probably over a million people are infected with the virus. Many of them do not know that they are infected; some do not even know that they are at risk, the female sexual partners of bisexual men being a good example. Even so, there is no sign that health professionals are being infected with the virus.

One special risk that does exist for health professionals is the 'needle-stick' injury, in which the professional is taking blood with a syringe and the needle slips and accidentally stabs the worker. Taking blood is not always easy and hospital staff are sometimes careless. In only one case has the health professional definitely been infected with the virus in this way, and in that case the nurse involved managed to micro-inoculate herself with a significant amount of infected blood. There have been two other probable cases via needle-sticks for which full details are not available. None of the three developed AIDS. In contrast, over 650 cases of needle-stick injury have been recorded involving HTLV-III infected blood in which there has been no sign of infection and there have probably been many more unreported needle-sticks in which nothing has happened. This underlines the low infectiousness of this virus.

The contrast with another virus, hepatitis B, is striking. There have been a number of cases now in which needle-stick injuries have occurred involving a patient who is dually infected with HTLV-III and hepatitis B, in several of which the health professional has been infected with hepatitis B but none of them was infected with HTLV-III. This is a much less infectious virus than hepatitis B.

Despite these considerations it makes sense to take precautions. A good example comes from dentistry. Far too few UK dentists take even simple precautions to protect themselves and their patients from infection. There is a lot of blood in dentistry and it is always sensible for a dentist to wear gloves, a mask and some form of eye protection when working. Even if these precautions are not vital from the point of view of HTLV-III infection, they are sensible clinical procedures and protect both the dentist and the patient.

Similarly, few health professionals wear gloves when taking blood but it would seem important that they should wear gloves for any invasive procedure. Again, even if HTLV-III presents no great risk in this respect, other things in blood do.

In fact one of the main causes of needle-stick injuries is

people re-sheathing needles when they have finished with them instead of simply dumping the whole lot in a 'sharps' box. It is easy to slip and impale onself and it is quite unnecessary.

HTLV-III underlines the fact that there needs to be a general tightening up of clinical procedures in hospitals. The precautions required are minimal. If the same precautions are taken as for hepatitis B infection there is no risk to anyone. The other important factor is that all patients need to be treated as potentially infected with HTLV-III. We have seen HTLV-III infected patients at every age from teenagers to people in their seventies and of both sexes. Some of these patients had absolutely no idea that they were at risk. Some were the sexual partners of bisexuals, others were men who had had isolated homosexual experiences but had been heterosexual for some time. There is no point in health staff relying on trying to identify those in high-risk groups and giving them special treatment. It is easy to fall into the trap of treating someone known to be infected with enormous care and then assuming that the person in the next bed is totally clear of infection and not bothering with precautions. An interesting illustration of this comes from laboratory practice. In the UK blood samples thought to be infected with some disease-causing organism are labelled with a 'biohazard' sticker and in many laboratories these are treated with enormous care. The stickers tend to encourage the quite incorrect assumption that those bloods which are not stickered must be perfectly safe: all too often they are sloshed about with something dangerously like contempt.

Nor can health professionals rely on testing to protect them. Firstly, up to 4% of results will be 'false negatives' and so one infected patient in 25 will not show up on the test. Secondly, the cost of testing every patient being admitted would bankrupt the average hospital. Thirdly, in view of the repercussions for the patient of being found positive on the test – not being able to get life insurance or an endowment mortgage, possibly not being able to change jobs, not to mention the personal cost – it would be necessary to inform the patient first that the test was going to be done and get their consent. It certainly would not be ethical not to do so and it might, depending on the circumstances, often not be legal either. Fourthly, there are many situations where testing is just not possible anyway. When an emergency operation is required it is hardly possible to wait a month for a set of test results.

The answer is, of course, straightforward. If all patients are treated with the same degree of care then no one need have any worries.

The silliest thing of all to do is to refuse to treat those patients who are seropositive. Far too many dentists and doctors in the UK and America have done this. It is short-sighted because all it will do is to lead to patients not telling their dentist or doctor that they are infected. The outcome of that will be a state of blissful ignorance for the practitioner but no net gain for anyone. And, of course, the care of the patients themselves may well suffer if useful clinical information is being kept from the doctor or dentist. Similarly, confidentiality for the patient is absolutely vital. AIDS is a sexually transmitted disease and for many men admitting they have it involves a double disclosure, not only that they are infected with a virus which is the subject of a national panic, but also that they are homosexual. If people think that there is any chance whatsoever that the information that they are infected with the virus will get out they will fail to seek treatment, with dire consequences. Confidentiality is guaranteed by law in the UK for all those having sexually transmitted diseases, as it is in some other European countries. Patients have a moral and a legal right to expect that information will not be passed on without their consent to third parties not involved directly in their treatment.

On a more global level, the costs of the current epidemic are likely to be huge. It probably costs £40,000 to treat an AIDS patient for a year, depending on the drugs being used and on how you calculate your costs. As the number of cases soars the amount of cash having to be diverted into this sort of work will rise sharply too. There is no doubt that governments will have to step in with more cash. Even in those countries where health care is on a mainly private basis it is likely that governments will have to underwrite at least part of the costs.

It is not only in the health services that there are likely to be problems. Community services are also likely to be stretched. When people become ill, particularly young people who have not built up reserves of money, they may not be able to work or to work to the same extent. The resulting financial problems lead to difficulties in housing and with bills. They may require additional services from the towns or cities in which they live in the form of help in the house or even deliveries of food ('meals on wheels'). One thing which might worsen the situation considerably is the encephalopathy which a proportion of HTLV-III infected people show. It is not just AIDS patients who show this sort of problem. In the worst cases it leads to a dementia-like illness. It is too early to say how common this sort of problem is likely to be, but the authors have seen quite a number of cases and other workers have reported it repeatedly. The prospect of even moderate numbers of young severely neurologically impaired people having to be cared for in hospital or in the community is appalling. There is simply no provision in most countries for long-term care of young people with this sort of problem.

Chapter Twelve

THE SEARCH FOR A CURE

The question everyone working in AIDS wants answered is, 'When will there be a cure?' Hardly surprisingly in the circumstances, patients often become terribly impatient with the apparently slow progress of research, and they sometimes worry that researchers are simply not putting enough effort into finding a cure: this is certainly not the case.

Many research groups throughout the world are looking at different approaches to the problem. It is an exciting challenge: the person who finds an answer will win fame and fortune (and deservedly so), the drug company which markets a cure will make big profits and the hospital or university which houses the successful team will acquire enormous prestige. There is another factor as well. Modern medicine can treat or prevent most infections, very few of which kill young men and women. So all clinicians are desperately keen to find a cure for AIDS and make their patients better. After all, that is why they are in the job in the first place.

There is currently a race on to find a cure for AIDS with institutions and researchers all over the world rushing to find the answer. More research money is, as always, needed: there is never enough money for research, always more you could do with a bit more cash. Even so, it is not money alone that matters, but also good ideas and luck. There are plenty of ideas, and we can only hope that there will be plenty of luck.

A cure for AIDS is not the only thing that matters, it is also important to find a way to prevent people who are infected with the virus going on to get AIDS, to stop the person who is infected being infectious to others, and, of course, to prevent someone who is not infected from becoming infected. Several ways are being tried at the moment.

DRUGS

The obvious weak link in the virus's progress is its use of reverse transcriptase. If a way could be found of blocking this enzyme, the virus would be unable to infect other cells and so it could not multiply within the patient's body. Several drugs have this action of blocking reverse transcriptase; for instance the French have been carrying out trials of a drug called HPA-23. Other workers have been experimenting with an old drug called suramin, originally developed for treating sleeping sickness.

The full results of trials with these drugs are not yet available, but there seems to be little evidence that they are likely to cure AIDS. The problem with reverse transcriptase blockers is likely to be that, although they may stop the virus replicating, they will probably not reverse the damage to the immune system which results in AIDS. It may be that they will prove more useful in preventing someone developing AIDS than in treating AIDS itself. It is also possible that they might be used in combination with methods aimed at boosting the immune system. This is discussed later.

The other problem with drugs like HPA-23 and suramin is that they can be toxic. This limits the amount of the drugs that can be given as well as the length of time that the drugs can be given for. It is also clearly not a good idea to give someone who is already sick a drug that is toxic if this can be at all avoided. Even if they prove to be able to keep the virus down, it may be that as soon as the drugs are discontinued the virus will start to make a come back. One particular worry is that the virus infects cells in the brain. Only a minority of drugs used in medicine actually cross into the brain, which has its own highly effective protective mechanisms against chemicals in the blood. Suramin, for instance, does not pass into the brain. Thus the brain could provide a reservoir of virus from which it might potentially spread again once the drug was stopped.

A lot of problems might be solved if a low toxicity reverse transcriptase blocker could be developed which could both cross into the brain and be used over a long period of time. It is also important to produce an oral drug, one that does not need to be injected, if it is to be taken over months or years. Drugs are being developed with these properties and they appear promising but we do not yet know how successful they will be.

This is, however, a very important area of research. One drug has been found in recent years which specifically treats herpes simplex virus infections and has made a great difference to the treatment of these infections. Although it has no action against HTLV-III, it does show that it is possible to develop drugs which attack specific viruses. There must be grounds for some degree of optimism about a successful drug being developed.

VACCINES

The first time you were exposed to measles you developed a characteristic rash and felt ill: fairly soon the measles resolved and you got better. Throughout their lives people will be exposed from time to time to the measles virus but not develop measles, because the immune system remembers that it has met the virus before and therefore does not have to start from scratch in fighting it. It is able to attack earlier and more effectively to prevent the virus getting a hold. In practice, special 'memory' B- and T-cells exist which are able to respond very rapidly to a second infection. This ability to respond earlier to a second attack than to a first is, of course, the reason why most infections are common in childhood but rare in adulthood. The young child is meeting most infections for the first time, the adult is protected from them.

One way to avoid being infected with a disease in the first place is to be vaccinated against it. The easiest way to see how this works is to look at an example. Smallpox has been eradicated from the world since 1977 as a result of isolation of cases and the use of a vaccine. The vaccine used is a virus called vaccinia, a close relative of the smallpox virus that does not itself cause smallpox. It is probably a variant of cowpox virus, which causes a smallpox-like infection in cattle. The immune system responds to vaccinia and eliminates the virus, and then the memory of having met the virus is retained by the immune system. Because vaccinia is so similar to smallpox virus, if the person meets smallpox virus the immune system recognises it and attacks it.

Smallpox is unusual in that a relatively harmless virus is so similar to it. In practice most vaccines have been made artificially. Most vaccines used today are either attenuated (weakened) versions of the virus against which they protect or 'killed' vaccines, which still possess the ability to stimulate the immune system, but not of course to cause disease. Recently, new ways of making vaccines have been developed. As discussed in Chapter 2, the immune system tends not to react to the whole of a virus particle but to a part, or sometimes several parts, of the virus. The part it responds to is called an antigen. In order to protect someone by vaccination only the antigen need be given to them. Since this is usually only a part of the virus it will not in itself cause disease.

This sounds fairly straightforward, but there are in practice a number of problems. Although the antigen may stimulate the immune system pretty well when it is part of the virus, it sometimes works less well on its own. For a variety of rather complex chemical reasons, antigens often stimulate the immune system best when they are stuck to other molecules. There have been two approaches to dealing with this. One approach has been to take a harmless virus and to build the antigen into it through genetic engineering. The harmless virus is then used as a vaccine and protects against the disease whose antigen it carries. The other approach is to build an artificial structure (called an iscom) which will present the antigen in such a way as to stimulate the immune system maximally and then to use the iscom as a vaccine.

Perhaps the best way to stop the AIDS epidemic would be to develop a vaccine against HTLV-III which could be given to anyone in a risk group. There are a number of special problems in developing a vaccine for HTLV-III. Firstly, it has no known safe relative which could be used in the same way as vaccinia with smallpox, so there is no easy vaccine option.

Vaccines work best where a virus is always the same. Measles is similar the world over, therefore the antigens it contains are always much the same, therefore measles vaccine always prevents infection. In contrast, it is very difficult to make a good general influenza vaccine. Influenza is caused by a group of viruses which from time to time mutate, that is, they change their structure sufficiently for the body no longer to recognise them. This is why there are periodic epidemics of influenza. What happens is straightforward. A new strain of 'flu appears and sweeps through the population. Many people catch it, they become ill, their immune systems fight it and they develop immunity to that strain of 'flu. After a few years the virus changes. People's immune systems are unable to recognise the new strain and once again the virus creates an epidemic. 'Flu vaccines can be developed, but they have to be developed for each new strain that appears.

HTLV-III seems to be more like 'flu and less like measles: it is a very variable virus. HTLV-III isolated from different people can vary in its genome by at least 7–8%, which is quite a lot. This makes developing a vaccine difficult, since a vaccine developed from virus taken from one person may not protect against virus that another person has. Some parts of the HTLV-III virus seem to be 'conserved', that is, consistent from person to person, and a vaccine would have to be aimed at these conserved areas.

The other problem is even more difficult to resolve. The body is able to fight measles effectively. The vaccine simply allows the body to prepare itself against something which will not cause the disease itself, thus preventing subsequent infection with measles. The body makes the same response to the vaccine as it would to measles itself. With HTLV-III the immune system seems unable to control the infection, at least not totally. For instance, the antibodies produced by the body in response to HTLV-III seem not to neutralise the virus effectively. Why this should be so is unclear, and we cannot be sure that antibodies produced to a vaccine would work any better. Therefore we do not know whether a vaccine would work at all.

There may be ways around this problem. Firstly, it may be that the virus is actually doing something to stop the antibodies working, therefore the vaccine might not have the problems of the real virus in stimulating a strong immune response. Secondly, it looks possible that some people may produce some effective antibody, but not enough actually to stop the virus. If a vaccine could be developed that would cause large amounts of such neutralising antibodies to be produced, it might prove effective. It is possible that an artificial vaccine might be built with these properties.

Several possible vaccines against HTLV-III are being developed at the moment. There must be grounds for optimism that a suitable vaccine will eventually be in general use.

IMMUNE STIMULATION

AIDS is really a partial failure of the immune system. If some way could be found to restore the immune system's functioning it might be possible to reverse the course of the disease. The difficulty, as always, is how this can be achieved.

One possibility is to take T-cells from someone who is healthy and transfuse them into someone with AIDS. There have been attempts to do this, but it has so far not proved as successful as was hoped. There are a number of technical difficulties with the process, but the real problem seems to be that the virus is able simply to infect the new T-cells in the same way as it infected the old. This suggests that it might at least be possible to combine immune stimulation with drugs blocking reverse transcriptase, if suitable drugs could be found.

Another possibility is to transplant tissue from the thymus, an organ which is very important in the development cycle of T-cells, which might improve the availability of mature T-cells in AIDS patients. Unfortunately, the evidence so far does not show that this procedure will be particularly effective. Again the problem seems to be the fact that the virus is able to attack new T-cells as soon as they are made, and some effort probably needs to be made to keep the virus at bay until a transplant can work.

Yet another possibility is to use a natural chemical called Interleukin-2. This makes T-cells more active and also makes them replicate in the laboratory. Either T-cells could be taken out of the patient, treated with Interleukin-2 and then put back, or Interleukin-2 could be used directly on the patient. The problem again is that anything which makes more T-cells available invites further infection of those T-cells with HTLV-III.

Another chemical that has been tried is interferon. There are several different kinds of interferon, each with rather different sorts of action. The interferons received much attention in the 1970s when the press hailed them as a possible cure for cancer, followed by mass disappointment when this proved not to be the case. In fact some interferons do have some effects against some types of cancer. Others play an important part in helping the body to resist virus infections. In AIDS the interferons have been used to treat Kaposi's sarcoma and other tumours, to try to prevent opportunistic infections, particularly viral ones, and to try to stimulate the immune system against HTLV-III. Results have been mixed and difficulties about dose, the type of interferon used and the source of the interferon have made the results difficult to interpret. Overall results have been rather disappointing. There is certainly no evidence that the interferons deal with the underlying infection in AIDS, or cure the immune deficiency, but they may sometimes help in treating tumours and keeping people free from opportunistic infections.

Before Fleming identified penicillin few people would have predicted that the infections which killed millions every year would soon be easily and effectively treated by antibiotics. Nor did hip replacement or organ transplants look possible at one time. Once a medical discovery has been made the steps leading up to it always seem easy and straightforward, even sometimes obvious. After all, various primitive tribes had used moulds to treat infected wounds for years before penicillin was identified – from a mould, but no one really took any notice.

A very large number of approaches to the treatment of HTLV-III infections are being tried at the moment. Although the information in this chapter may seem discouraging, there are certainly grounds for optimism: no one can tell what is just around the corner. After all, the virus itself was only identified in 1983 and the progress in understanding it has been phenomenal in the short time that has elapsed since then.

Chapter Thirteen

THE FUTURE

Nothing can make someone look so foolish so fast as a prediction, but it is always interesting to speculate, always helpful to plan, and making plans means making guesses.

In the USA the number of AIDS cases has been doubling roughly every eight to ten months. There are some signs that this may be slowing, to double in perhaps twelve to eighteen months. It may be that part of this slowing is the result of people becoming slower to report cases and part of it a real change. Either way, it must be remembered that the disease is still on the increase: only the rate of increase is changing.

The number of people infected in the USA is hard to guess: it may be as high as a million. In Britain there may be 20,000 at the time of writing, with the numbers climbing sharply. In the UK and Europe the number of cases is still doubling every six to eight months with no signs of slowing. The people infected at the moment are mainly in high-risk groups. Because there are only a limited number of people in high-risk groups, the steeply climbing curve of new infections and new cases will eventually level off. No one knows how many cases there will be when it does so.

The only thing that would stop it levelling off is if the infection becomes common among heterosexuals. There are far more heterosexuals than homosexuals, so the virus would get a new lease of life. No one really knows whether the virus is going to spread widely among heterosexuals. There are several ways that it could. It could spread because so many men are bisexual and because many men are homosexual in their teens and early twenties and then shift towards heterosexual behaviour. Because it is a recent infection we probably have not yet seen the effects of this to any great extent. It could spread out from intravenous drug abusers on the back of one of the other great health problems of our time.

The proportion of AIDS cases in the USA who are heterosexual has not changed greatly over the last two years. That may be reassuring, or it may only reflect the lag between people becoming infected and developing AIDS. Or it may be that heterosexuals have fewer co-factors, other infections which may promote AIDS in someone who is infected with the virus. Heterosexual cases of HTLV-III infection may simply be less likely to be identified. Many women, in particular, may not know that their husband is bisexual and thus not come forward for testing. It may simply reflect the lag which is likely before the virus spreads out from the groups it first infected.

HTLV-III infection currently has a low base among heterosexuals. Not many people are infected and, on average, heterosexuals tend to have fewer partners than gay men. Taking into account the crossover between the gay and heterosexual populations, any spread is likely to be slow at the moment. If the numbers once built up beyond a certain point the infection would, however, really take off.

The example of Africa is something of a warning. There the disease is a heterosexually spread one. There are special factors in Africa, the high rate of usage of prostitutes probably being the main one. We do not of course know what the rate of usage of prostitutes is in the West. But the African experience does show two things, that this is a disease which can easily be spread heterosexually and that once the virus gets a big hold it soon runs completely out of control.

No one knows what will happen. It is likely that there will be a slow spread among heterosexuals over the next few years. Whether the acceleration will then happen depends on a number of factors that are difficult to calculate, in part because even less is known about the current sexual behaviour of heterosexuals than that of gay men. Undoubtedly the use of condoms by heterosexuals for casual sex would limit the degree of spread considerably. There is time for heterosexuals to put such measures into practice, but there is a question mark over whether they will indeed take these steps.

Intravenous drug abusers are likely to be a major disaster area in the next two or three years. HTLV-III infection levels among heroin addicts have already reached epidemic proportions in America, up to 80% in parts of New York. All the signs are that in Britain and throughout Europe exactly the same thing is happening. In some areas of Britain today up to 50% of heroin users attending clinics are infected, compared with perhaps 1–2% only two years ago. Only the most determined health education campaign stands any chance of defeating the problem. There are two problems to be dealt with, the alarming rise in drug abuse which is afflicting virtually every Western country and for which there seems to be at the moment no obvious solution, and the spread of HTLV-III among intravenous drug abusers, for which the answer is to dissuade them from sharing syringes. Unfortunately there is every sign that the two problems are tangled up in the minds of governments, and sometimes of clinicians working in the field. They need to get them untangled pretty rapidly if anything is to be done before it is too late.

The only bright area is that blood transfusions and blood products should be safe from now on and that the number of haemophiliacs being infected for the first time should be reduced, it is hoped to none.

For governments the problem of HTLV-III will create a tremendous burden. The extra medical facilities to cope with AIDS cases and the increased demand for facilities in the community will not come cheap. If HTLV-III turns out to produce brain damage on any sort of scale, the other costs will pale into insignificance compared with the expense of looking after numbers of young neurologically impaired patients, something for which there is virtually no provision in any Western country today.

The spread of the virus may also have great social impact. It is doubtful that society is likely to move back to Victorian morality – always more illusory than real in any case. Nor would such a change be desirable, since it was based largely on ignorance and hypocrisy. However, both heterosexuals and homosexuals are likely to find that their sexual freedoms carry more of a price than they have in the past. Certainly the signs are that those gay men who have had many partners in the past are reducing their number of partners. If the virus starts to spread widely amongst heterosexuals a similar pattern will probably result there also. The condom is likely to make a major come-back, in the role that it had in Victorian and Georgian times of a protection against sexually transmitted diseases, rather than as a contraceptive.

With no cure for AIDS and a vaccine perhaps five years or more away, there is little medical that can be done at the moment to stop the spread of the disease. The only thing that can be done now is to persuade people whose behaviour puts them at risk to change their behaviour to reduce that risk. That means health education, which must be backed up with facilities for people actually to meet counsellors, whether via voluntary organisations or in hospitals and clinics, and get advice on how to put the necessary changes into practice. It is fine to publish posters and leaflets about safer sex, but the changes in sexual behaviour that people must make are enormous and the difficulty of putting them into practice should not be underestimated. It often helps to talk over the problems with someone who understands the situation and can offer concrete advice.

In the same way, it is vital to persuade intravenous drug users to use clean syringes and not to share them. Just putting out posters in drug clinics is unlikely to help: there must be a concrete effort to reach those drug users who are on the street and are not coming into contact with clinics, certainly by far the majority. It is also a waste of time advising drug users to use a clean syringe unless they can get one fairly easily. It is doubtful that the average drug user has the motivation to search out twenty pharmacies in order to find one that might let him have a syringe.

HTLV-III is spreading widely, and so are its relatives HTLV-I and HTLV-II, at least amongst American gay men. While it seems unlikely that these will present the problems of HTLV-III, they may well become problems of their own.

The only silver lining in this particular cloud seems to be that the arrival of HTLV-III has concentrated massive research on other medical puzzles. Could some of those be the result of viral infections, perhaps with retroviruses, perhaps with other viruses? Much investigation is going on at the moment into a whole range of other illnesses. In solving the problem of HTLV-III it is just possible that we may be able to solve some of the other mysteries of medicine. And if an HTLV-V and an HTLV-VI are waiting in the wings, as they could well be, we may be better prepared next time. It is slim comfort, but it is perhaps something.

Appendix

USEFUL ADDRESSES FOR HIGH-RISK GROUPS

Body Positive. A resource and support organisation for those who are HTLV-III seropositive.
Address: Body Positive, BM AIDS, London WC1N 3XX

The Terrence Higgins Trust. A registered charity providing face-to-face and telephone counselling, support groups and 'buddy' services for those with AIDS, and an information service for those with AIDS-related worries.
Address: Terrence Higgins Trust, BM AIDS, London WC1N 3XX
Telephone Help Line: 01-833 2971 (7.00–10.00 p.m., Mon.–Fri.)

London Lesbian and Gay Switchboard. A telephone advisory, counselling and referral service for gay people and for those with health-related concerns, run completely by gay people.
Telephone: 01-837 7324 (24 hours daily, year round)

Haemophilia Society. Information, research and advisory service for haemophiliacs and their families.
Address: PO Box 9, 16 Trinity Street, London SE1 1DE
Telephone: 01-407 1010

Health Education Council
   Address: 78 Oxford Street, London WC1A 1AH
   Telephone: 01-631 0930

From Miller, D., Weber, J., Green, J. (eds), *The Management of AIDS Patients*. London: Macmillan Press, 1986.

INDEX

147